Praise for H. Robert Superko, M.D., and *Before the Heart Attacks*

"An understanding of the classic risk factors is still essential, but it seems clear that we are entering a new phase in the quest for heart health. And cardiologist Robert Superko is one of those leading the way . . . *Before the Heart Attacks* offers a comprehensive guide to the latest ideas in preventing coronary heart disease."   —*Newsweek*

"Looks beyond people with obvious risk factors to those who will become victims of 'unexpected' heart attacks, noting that half of all attacks occur in people with normal cholesterol levels. It feels evangelistic but not preachy, comprehensive . . . but not forbidding."—*The Washington Post*

"[Superko] is a man at the center of the cardiac establishment promoting nothing less than a total makeover of diagnosis and treatment. His central claim is remarkable. His findings are set out in a new book . . . which everyone with cardiac concerns should read."
—*The Times* (London)

H. Robert Superko, M.D., is cofounder of the prestigious Berkeley Heart Lab in California. He has published over one hundred scientific articles in top journals, including the *New England Journal of Medicine* and the *Journal of the American Medical Association,* and is a frequent speaker at American College of Cardiology meetings. He is currently director of the Cholesterol, Genetics, and Heart Disease Institute in Burlingame, California, and the medical director for progressive arteriosclerosis management at the Fuqua Heart Center at Piedmont Hospital in Atlanta, Georgia. He lives in Portola Valley, California.

Laura Tucker is the coauthor of several health and medical books. She lives in Brooklyn, New York.

This book results from the work of many dedicated scientists, nurses, nutritionists, and physicians who have searched for the answers to the puzzle of heart disease for more than 50 years. They are too numerous to single out, but one in particular needs to be mentioned. Dr. John Gofman, at the University of California, Berkeley, discovered the importance of different types of LDLs and HDLs for heart health more than 50 years ago and was decades ahead of his time.

The book is dedicated to two young men and all their counterparts: my two sons, Scott and Alex, and all the other children with a history of coronary heart disease in their families. Although Alex and Scott undoubtedly carry some of my family's heart disease genes, the knowledge we have discovered, and will discover soon, creates a much brighter future for them. They have suffered to some degree from their father's obsession with fighting this disease through his frequent absences required by scientific research meetings, lectures, meetings for the American Heart Association and American College of Cardiology, and yes, writing commitments such as this book. But perhaps in some small way they have benefited. As strange as it may sound, I find joy in and fascination with cholesterol, and by sharing this joy and fascination and helping to solve a part of the heart disease puzzle with Alex and Scott, I hope to encourage them to find their own passion in life and not be discouraged if at some point they are criticized for being ahead of the curve. This book is also dedicated to my father and mother.

My personal experience that led me on this path first involved my father, Harold Robert Superko Sr., a Navy captain, who was a victim of premature heart disease, and my mother, Earlene M. Superko, who died in my arms as a result of the ravages of this disease. My father died suddenly from his second heart attack when I was a young medical student, and at the time I was puzzled that we, the medical community, could not answer exactly why he had the disease. He came from a coal mining family in Nanticoke, Pennsylvania, and rose to be a captain in the United States Navy dental corps. He was not fat, did not smoke, followed a reasonable diet, and was not identified as a person at high risk for heart attack. Later, while training in the coronary care unit at the University of California, Davis, it also puzzled me that we spent a tremendous amount of time and money putting out the fires of acute heart attacks, but once the patients left the unit, we gave them almost no advice on what caused their disease or how to aggressively attack it. Instead of pursuing a typical cardiology career I felt compelled to do as much as possible to help discover the causes of this terrible disease, which would then lead to individualized treatments to prevent others from suffering the fate of my father and mother.

—H. Robert Superko, M.D.

BEFORE THE HEART ATTACKS

H. **ROBERT SUPERKO**, M.D., F.A.C.C., F.A.H.A.

WITH LAURA TUCKER

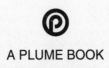

A PLUME BOOK

PUBLISHER'S NOTE
Every effort has been made to ensure that the information contained in this book is complete and accurate. However, neither the publisher nor the author is engaged in rendering professional advice or services to the individual reader. The ideas, procedures, and suggestions contained in this book are not intended as a substitute for consulting with your physician. All matters regarding your health require medical supervision. Neither the author nor the publisher shall be liable or responsible for any loss or damage allegedly arising from any information or suggestion in this book.

Beginning on page 283, you will find safe-use guidelines for supplements recommended in this book that will help you use these remedies safely and wisely.

Mention of specific companies, organizations, or authorities in this book does not imply endorsement by the publisher, nor does mention of specific companies, organizations, or authorities imply that they endorse this book. Internet addresses and telephone numbers given in this book were accurate at the time it went to press.

PLUME
Published by the Penguin Group
Penguin Group (USA) Inc., 375 Hudson Street, New York, New York 10014, U.S.A.
Penguin Books Ltd, 80 Strand, London WC2R 0RL, England
Penguin Books Australia Ltd, 250 Camberwell Road, Camberwell, Victoria 3124, Australia
Penguin Books Canada Ltd, 10 Alcorn Avenue,Toronto, Ontario, Canada M4V 3B2
Penguin Books India (P) Ltd, 11 Community Centre, Panchsheel Park, New Delhi–110 017, India
Penguin Books (NZ), cnr Airborne and Rosedale Roads, Albany, Auckland 1310, New Zealand
Penguin Books (South Africa) (Pty) Ltd, 24 Sturdee Avenue,
Rosebank, Johannesburg 2196, South Africa

Penguin Books Ltd, Registered Offices: 80 Strand, London WC2R 0RL, England

Published by Plume, a member of Penguin Group (USA) Inc. This is an authorized reprint of a hardcover edition published by Rodale Inc. For information address Rodale Inc., 733 Third Avenue, 15th Floor, New York, NY 10017-3204.

First Plume Printing, June 2004
10 9 8 7 6 5 4 3 2

Ⓟ REGISTERED TRADEMARK—MARCA REGISTRADA

The Library of Congress has catalogued the Rodale edition as follows:

Superko, H. Robert.
    Before the heart attacks : a revolutionary approach to detecting,
preventing, and even reversing heart disease / H. Robert Superko, with
Laura Tucker ; with forewords by Spencer B. King III and Harvey S. Hecht.
        p.   cm.
    Includes bibliographical references and index.
    ISBN 1–57954–800–8 (hc.)
    ISBN 0-452-28526-7 (pbk.)
    1. Coronary heart disease—Prevention—Popular works.   I. Tucker,
Laura.   II. Title.
RC685.C6S79   2003
616.1'2305—dc21   2003007401

Printed in the United States of America

CONTENTS

BEFORE
THE
HEART
ATTACKS

FOREWORD

HEART ATTACK IS THE LEADING CAUSE OF DEATH in the developed world. I have been caring for patients with coronary heart disease for over 30 years, and during the course of my career I have consistently heard the same questions. What causes a heart attack? How can I prevent one? What are my prospects after a heart attack? I have noticed in recent years, however, that my patients are beginning to ask more sophisticated questions. They want to know more specifically what is wrong and why. How do arteries become blocked? What are the factors that cause the arteries to become diseased? Have I inherited a condition that is putting me at risk? What about my children: Should I be concerned? What tests are needed to identify my risks? Can I modify these risk factors? If so, will that prevent a heart attack?

Dr. Robert Superko, a leading scientist at the forefront of cardiac research, has focused his work on the question of how to *prevent* heart attacks. In *Before the Heart Attacks* he has now distilled his extensive clinical experience with a wealth of scientific studies to offer patients, and those wishing to *avoid* becoming patients, answers to these and many other questions. He is able to present in a compelling and thoroughly understandable way the science behind what goes wrong in coronary heart disease as well as recent breakthroughs in cardiac care. This book enables the general reader to understand and be able to improve his or her own odds.

For years, Dr. Superko and many other scientists have uncovered the basic mechanisms by which arteries deposit fat, become inflamed, and clot. These mechanisms are not the same for all people, and they are frequently complex. Simply prescribing statin drugs is not the answer for everyone! Many have tried to simplify the complex with unfortunate results. Dr. Superko instead recognizes the full complexity but succeeds in breaking it down for readers so that they can understand their own specific metabolic makeup and seek the solutions that are right for them. This book explains how heart attacks can be averted, from lifestyle changes to drug therapies to modifications of the effects of an individual's genes.

Those who read this book can be assured that they are not getting just another opinion or theory, but the most up-to-date findings backed by the scientific evidence underlying our most important disease. Some will find the answers right here; all will leave this book empowered to ask the questions necessary to lead them to those answers.

Spencer B. King III, M.D., M.A.C.C.

Fuqua Chair of Interventional Cardiology, The Fuqua Heart Center at Piedmont Hospital;
The American Cardiovascular Research Institute; clinical professor of medicine, Emory
University School of Medicine; former president, American College of Cardiology

March 2003

PREFACE

OUR BEST EFFORTS NOTWITHSTANDING, the medical community hasn't made much of an impact in preventing coronary heart disease. For 150,000 people every year the first symptom of heart disease is the last: a fatal heart attack. Every year more than 1 million people experience heart attacks, and if they survive, will very likely not be provided with the tools to prevent a second episode.

So, what is the answer? A significant contribution to the imperative goal of preventing both first and subsequent heart attacks is provided in this book by Dr. Robert Superko.

This is an age of empowerment, particularly in health care. At no time in history has the public been so aware of the latest trends. Our patients read about the newest advances in the newspaper before they are published in scientific journals. Unfortunately, most of what occupies the media's fancy vanishes quickly, having neither the scientific validity nor the ability to impact a significant number of lives. But the science that Dr. Superko is popularizing in this book is of supreme interest to both physicians and their patients.

All snowflakes are, by definition, snowflakes, yet no two are alike. Similarly, we are all human (although some would argue differently), yet no two are identical. Even identical twins, by interacting differently with the environment, may have quite different cardiac health despite their identical genetic makeup. These two principles, i.e., the uniqueness of every individual and the ability to alter our genetically determined fate, are an essential part of Dr. Superko's concepts. The ability to characterize our patients' metabolic risks through the advanced lipid testing, followed by alteration of that risk by recommending individual drug, diet, and exercise programs, offers a significant advance over conventional approaches. Moreover, it facilitates a true partnership between the physician and the patient who can work together in an interactive relationship.

We are all creatures of habit, particularly physicians, who, for a multiplicity of reasons, tend to think in repetitive patterns based upon conventional models. However, significant advances rarely occur by following the status quo. But going above and beyond requires the insight to recognize the right ideas, the scientific justification for their implementation, and the courage to pursue them despite sometimes vigorous opposition. For the past 10 years, I have been a witness to, and a participant in, Dr. Superko's journey. We have collaborated in the care of numerous patients and in scientific investigations and publications. I have incorporated his principles into the new field of "interventional lipidology," which combines the identification of risk through the remarkable power of calcified plaque imaging by electron beam tomography, with the identification and treatment of the metabolic factors responsible for that risk as described in this volume.

The concepts embodied in *Before the Heart Attacks* will ultimately be accepted as being obvious and will be universally implemented. Readers of this volume will have the privilege of reaping its benefits to prolong their own lives, and by incorporating the principles described in great yet eminently readable detail, can extend the benefits to family members of the present and future generations. I will certainly be recommending it to all my patients and believe that this book should also be required reading for all doctors dedicated to making substantial gains in our preventive battle against heart disease.

Harvey S. Hecht, M.D., F.A.C.C.
Director of preventive cardiology, Beth Israel Medical Center,
Continuum Heart Institute, New York City
March 2003

ACKNOWLEDGMENTS

A GROUP OF HEALTH PROFESSIONALS who receive far too little credit are nutritionists. I would like to mention one in particular who helped tremendously with this book. Lisa Sawrey-Kubicek, M.S., R.D., has worked with me at Stanford University, the University of California, and Berkeley HeartLab. Her understanding of the science that surrounds nutrition and the advanced metabolic tests has allowed me to serve my patients much better, and she brings a breath of clarity to a field that is often confusing. She is responsible for the success of the nutrition aspects of this book.

As an author of many scientific articles and textbook chapters, and editor of scientific journals, I appreciate the difficult and often thankless job of editing. For this reason I would like to thank Laura Tucker, who was able to take my thoughts and perspective on this medical science and convert them from a rather complicated tome into something that is a pleasure to read. She was also able to do this in a remarkably short period of time.

The exercise, heart disease, and HDL cholesterol field would not be nearly this advanced if it were not for my friend and colleague Dr. Peter Wood. He is the scientist who discovered that HDL cholesterol is high in runners, in large part because he has been a lifelong long-distance runner himself and an observant scientist. Believe it or not, he made the observation about HDL cholesterol in runners while working on his own blood as a young scientist in Oakland, California. In subsequent years he conducted much of the National Institutes of Health research that clarified the effect of exercise and weight loss on HDL cholesterol and its subfractions.

—H. Robert Superko, M.D.

I WOULD LIKE TO THANK Dr. Robert Superko for his efforts to make this science accessible and available to the rest of the world; Richard and Leslie Curtis, for everything (per usual); and Carol Colman, for the opportunity. I'd also like to thank everyone at the Berkeley HeartLab, especially Anabey Camarena and Elaine Raul; the Diet Team: Christina Bilheimer, Kathy Hanuschak, and Lisa Sawrey-Kubicek; and the people at Rodale for their incredible professionalism, especially Kathy Dvorsky, Chris Krogermeier, Dan Listwa, and Deanna Portz. Endless love and thanks to my wonderful husband, Doug.

Much gratitude is due to Jeremy Katz for his patience, continued faith, and terrific advice throughout this project. And finally, I'd like to recognize Laurie Bernstein—my "other midwife"—for her friendship, knowledge, and genuinely heroic efforts on behalf of this book. Thanks are not enough: It truly could not have been done without her.

—Laura Tucker

INTRODUCTION

JOHN WAS IN TERRIFIC PHYSICAL CONDITION and the envy of all his friends, even some that were far younger than he. A marathon runner in his twenties and thirties, he was still running 25 miles a week at 54. His diet was exemplary: low fat, low calorie, low sodium, and his cholesterol levels and blood pressure were gorgeous. Yet after a bout of chest pains during a routine morning run took him into the emergency room, tests revealed that he would require an immediate quadruple bypass. Indeed, the surgeon who performed the operation said that, given the severity of his condition, it was a miracle John had survived as long as he had.

John's is the perfect example of the "stealth" heart attack, the one that no one sees coming. Every major cardiac event is frightening and traumatic, both for the patient and for his loved ones, but there is an additional layer of disbelief and horror attached when it happens to someone who had no reason to suspect he was even at risk.

For the moment, let's leave aside the seriously overweight and those who participate in behaviors like smoking that are known to put us at risk for coronary heart disease, as well as people who ignore or defy their doctor's ministrations, or who neglect themselves and fail to go for regular physicals.

Let us stay focused, for the moment, on those model individuals who are conscientious and health minded and who follow their doctor's advice—the ones who get all the recommended screening tests and who, despite their clean bills of health, still fall victim to a major and totally unexpected coronary event.

These "surprise" heart attacks are actually not rare at all. They are far more prevalent than any of us would, or *should*, be comfortable with.

There are an average of 1.5 million heart attacks in the United States each year. One-half of these strike people with "normal" cholesterol levels. That's right. A full 50 percent of the beds in acute cardiac care units are filled by patients who had none of the traditional red flags to warn of pending cardiac trouble. More shocking still, 80 percent of people who suffer heart attacks have the *same* cholesterol levels as people who don't suffer heart attacks!

Why is there no warning? How can coronary heart disease be so severe as to cause a heart attack—death, even—but not show up on our routine screening tests?

THE FALSE SUMMIT

Anyone who has ever climbed a mountain knows the thrill, after a long and arduous hike, of finally seeing and then reaching the crest. Achieving the summit erases the memory of the long hours, the hard work, the blisters. The view from the top makes it all worthwhile.

But there's another experience familiar to the seasoned hiker: You strain for those final yards against screaming muscles and a rebelling brain, and finally you pull yourself up to the top—only to discover that you've hit a false summit. The only reward of this new vantage point is that you are now able to see yet another, higher summit, some distance beyond the place where you are now standing. As you look up at this whole new mountain, you realize with dismay that you're only at the base of your final climb.

Back when researchers first discovered the correlation between cholesterol levels and heart disease, everyone thought that we'd discovered the root cause of coronary heart disease. We thought that doctors were finally in a position to intervene and save patients from a deadly and pernicious disease.

Those on the front line at the time felt on top of the world, or at least on top of the summit they had been scaling for so many years.

The mistake those researchers made was to believe that their cholesterol breakthrough meant they'd achieved the summit. They believed they had the problem licked, but in truth there was more road ahead. I know, because I was one of those researchers.

In fact, I participated in one of the original studies to determine the effects of lowering cholesterol on heart disease risk. Over the course of the study, we met with patients periodically to check in with them and to review their progress. Since that study included only male participants, I was surprised one afternoon to see a woman waiting for me. Her question to me was simple: "My husband's cholesterol numbers were perfect, and you told him that based on those numbers he was at low risk for heart disease. So why did he drop dead suddenly of a massive heart attack?"

As you can imagine, I was devastated, but at the time I didn't have an answer to give her. More than 20 years have passed since that day, and I now believe that I can finally offer her—and the many others who have lost a loved one to an unexpected heart attack—an answer to that question. In part, I write this book for that woman in my waiting room, and for everyone who has lost someone they love to this disease.

It's certainly true that the correlation between heart disease and cholesterol was a discovery of critical importance and great magnitude, and the standard cholesterol test—total cholesterol, LDL, HDL, and triglycerides—became (and remains) routine at every physical. Our mistake was in thinking that these tests gave us everything we needed to predict coronary heart disease and to effectively treat those at risk.

In fact, getting a good cholesterol "score" can actually have an injurious effect on your health. If you happen to have one of the 8 out of 10 disorders contributing to coronary heart disease that don't get caught by the standard tests, then getting a good score can lull you into a false sense of complacency, making you *think* that you're low risk—when you're really not. That means people who should be alert and vigilant won't take the precautions they should—and that people who *should* be treated won't be.

Conversely, some of the people who are found to be at high risk through these standard screening tests will seek and receive treatment for their high cholesterol. Many of those same individuals will later discover (often as they're being wheeled into the operating room) that high cholesterol wasn't the only culprit behind their cardiac disease.

Today we can finally explain how so many cases of coronary heart disease could have fallen through the cracks, causing sudden heart attacks in people thought to be low risk. In truth, these individuals *weren't* at low risk— they only appeared to be, because we were gauging risk by looking at only one piece of the total puzzle. We were missing a slew of additional red flags because we didn't yet know to look for them. We now know, for example, that 80 percent of all coronary heart disease is linked to genetic causes—yet the standard cholesterol tests are not designed to screen for even the most common genetic indicators.

THE NEW MARKERS THAT CAN PREDICT YOUR CARDIAC FUTURE

The standard cholesterol tests, while still an important and necessary step in screening for heart disease, are just the *first* step in determining your risk. We now know that we need also to look for a host of other factors—and it is from this more complete, composite picture that we are now able to predict with far greater accuracy your true cardiac risk.

The good news is that we are now able to go *beyond* cholesterol. Today we have the research and the technological capabilities to screen for a far broader spectrum of risk factors.

In particular, groundbreaking new research allows us to screen for a series of *metabolic markers*, indicators that sound an alarm to those trained in this new science. These markers give us an extremely sophisticated analysis, one that is far more sensitive, precise, and personalized than the information we can get from cholesterol tests alone. These tests pinpoint with exacting precision the underlying metabolic imbalances that could be putting you at risk for cardiovascular disease or heart attack. They allow us to predict, with a higher degree of reliability, the degree of cardiac risk you're actually facing. And with our new ability to detect and isolate these threats comes the power to launch a strategic and effective counteroffensive.

Diagnosing these Advanced Metabolic Markers allows us to fill in a final piece of information in your composite risk profile, what I call your Cardiac Fingerprint.

Your Cardiac Fingerprint is the summation of all the pertinent information about you and your heart: your family history of coronary heart disease, your lifestyle choices, your genetic predispositions, medical conditions, and any physical traits that might be putting you at risk for coronary heart disease. This Cardiac Fingerprint gives you and your doctor a truly reliable and comprehensive assessment tool for determining your present and future cardiac health status. Once we know specifically what's putting you at risk, it is also possible to counter with a more precise, individualized remedy.

Rest assured: No matter what information your Cardiac Fingerprint holds, we now have the power to change your cardiac destiny. Whether nature dealt you a tough hand or you've simply made some lifestyle choices over the years that have landed you in the danger zone, we can now guide you to programs that will help you to stop—if not reverse—the progression of your disease.

It is now possible to be treated *before* the heart attacks, while noninvasive measures can still effectively be employed to prevent and even reverse cardiovascular disease.

ONE SIZE DOES NOT FIT ALL

The true cornerstone of the new cardiology lies in the ability it gives us to customize care for each person. One size never did fit all and certainly not in cardiac care!

Have you ever wondered why some people respond beautifully to treatment, while others undergoing the same treatment for the same problem find that their efforts prove futile no matter what kind of dietary and drug hoops they jump through? Chances are, they're jumping through the wrong hoops. How frustrating for these patients, and how discouraging for their doctors!

The flaws inherent in a one-size-fits-all approach to cardiac care is apparent when we look at the basic low-fat, high-carbohydrate diet that's prescribed across the board for people with high cholesterol. Don't get me wrong: This is a very good diet for some people. But it's not good for everyone. Indeed, we now know that, depending upon what your markers reveal, this diet could actually be *detrimental* to your cardiac health.

This book is designed to help you find the *right* exercise, diet, and medication plans to fit *your specific* needs. The chapters that follow will guide you through the process of building the custom-fit program for your particular cardiac risk profile—an individualized set of Prescriptions that will finally deliver the results you have been working so hard to achieve. Stop blaming yourself; no amount of elbow grease can get the wrong key to turn in a lock. It's time to try a new key. Once you get the right fit, you'll get terrific results, and with a fraction of the effort.

The day of one-size-fits-all cardiac care is over; the purpose of this book is to show you what lies ahead. My hope is that this book will help to empower you to partner with your doctor in order to take control of your cardiac future.

HOW TO USE THIS BOOK

The first step, and part 1 of the book, is designed to help you put together your own Cardiac Fingerprint. Your Fingerprint is a true and accurate assessment of your risk status, including the inherited factors, genetic predispositions, physical traits, and lifestyle factors that, taken together, make up your current cardiac profile.

You'll begin that process in chapter 3 by filling out your Personal Risk Profile. This self-assessment quiz is the first step in discovering your true level of risk. We'll talk about cholesterol—only part of the picture, but an important part. And then you'll learn all about the groundbreaking new screening tests that can reveal for the first time, through a simple, inexpensive blood test, the Advanced Metabolic Markers that complete your Cardiac Fingerprint.

The self-assessment quizzes in the first part of the book will help you and your doctor to determine your level of risk, which in turn determines how aggressive your program should be. The next step, and part 2 of the book, will be to show you how to apply the information from your Cardiac Fingerprint to build an individualized treatment plan, custom-fit to your cardiac profile.

In chapters 7 through 10, you'll be led through the four legs of cardiac treatment: nutrition, exercise, medication, and supplements. Each section will offer some basics on the topic at hand, so that you'll understand what role it plays in cardiac health and how each one factors into your ability to take charge of your cardiac destiny. In these chapters, you'll plug your own Advanced Metabolic Marker results into the Prescription Keys, which will then guide you to the appropriate Plans as you build your individualized program. Each piece of the program will be matched specifically to your individual cardiac profile.

In the end you'll have a comprehensive health plan as unique as your Cardiac Fingerprint. Even those of you who haven't taken the advanced screening tests will be guided to specific diet and exercise programs, designed to start you on the road to cardiac health. No matter what your current cardiac status, this book can help show you the way to a heart-healthier life, starting today.

These recent advances in the field of cardiology now allow us to lay claim to the summit that once eluded us. Whether this is the last and final summit, I will not speculate—after cholesterol, I know better. I keep the epigraph from the 18th-century samurai that opens this chapter on my office wall as a constant reminder that a warrior cannot afford to become overconfident. When you are in battle against a foe as formidable as coronary heart disease, you must always assume that what you know is not enough.

Of this much I am certain: The groundbreaking strides we have recently made in the field, the strides that are the subject of this book, have the power to save countless lives and to change the face of cardiac care. I write this book to bring news of these momentous advancements and to explain what they mean for every single person who suffers from cardiac disease, believes they might be at risk, or loves someone who is.

We have now the opportunity to bring coronary heart disease to its knees, to make every heart attack an anomaly. I invite you to join me in outwitting your genetic destiny.

PART 1

DECODING YOUR CARDIAC FINGERPRINT

"A MAN IS ONLY AS OLD AS HIS ARTERIES."

—Sir William Osler,
The Principles and Practice of Medicine, 1892

1

HOW THE HEART WORKS AND HOW IT BREAKS

I'M ALWAYS A LITTLE SURPRISED when I discover just how little my patients, even ones with serious cardiovascular disease, actually know about the way their hearts work. So before we jump ahead to talk about specific risk, detection, and treatment measures, let's take a quick look at how every heart works and how its function is affected and impeded by disease.

THE HEART OF THE MATTER

This pump in the center of our chests truly is the source of life, and its importance is reflected in our poetry, our songs, our metaphors—in our very sense of who we are. Medieval scientists believed that the heart was the center of wisdom (true love, incidentally, was consigned to the liver). Today, we think of our heart as the center of our souls, the part that governs how we feel. When a love affair ends, we say our heart is broken. When someone acts in a humane way, we say his heart is in the right place. When we're speaking sincerely, our words are said to come from the heart. When we desperately want something, we say our heart is set on it. And when we suffer a great sadness, doesn't it feel like there's a heavy weight in precisely that region of our chest?

It's little wonder that this fist-size muscle is such an inspiration to us. The heart is truly a miraculous organ, even to someone who has studied it for as long as I have. An adult heart beats about 70 times a minute, which adds up to a staggering 100,000 times a day—and 2.5 *billion* times over the course of the average lifetime. The tube that eventually becomes the heart begins beating about 23 days after conception and keeps going until it stops for good.

The heart is divided into four chambers, or rooms: the **left atrium**, the **right atrium**, the **left ventricle**, and the **right ventricle**. Each chamber is sealed by a valve, so that blood can go one way but not the other. When you listen to a heartbeat, you can hear that the beat happens in two parts: *lub-dub*. The first part of the beat pushes the blood from the **atria** (the small chambers on the top of the heart) to the **ventricles** (the larger ones on the bottom), and the second part of the beat pushes the blood out of the heart.

Every single cell in our bodies requires oxygen to produce energy from food. It is the one essential ingredient; we cannot survive for any extended period of time without oxygen. This is why the heart is so important. Its primary job is to circulate oxygen-rich blood throughout our entire body. The two sides of the heart perform two different functions toward this end. The right side of the heart collects oxygen-poor blood and sends it to the lungs to be replenished with oxygen and to rid itself of carbon dioxide. The left side takes the oxygen-rich blood coming from the lungs and recirculates it through the body to your muscles and organs. Oxygenated (oxygen-rich) blood is carried by the arteries away from the heart, and oxygen-depleted blood is carried by the veins back to the heart.

HOW THE HEART BREAKS

Coronary heart disease is the leading cause of death in the United States. It can be caused by many different factors, including congenital heart defects, heart valve infections, and heartbeat irregularities. Throughout this book, we're going to be focusing primarily on **coronary artery disease** (CAD), which is the most common form of heart disease, affecting 7 million Americans today.

What is coronary artery disease?

Like all the cells and muscles in the body, the heart muscle itself needs oxygen. And as with the rest of the body, that life-sustaining oxygen is carried to the individual cells of the heart by arteries. These are called the **coronary arteries**. There are three main coronary arteries: one on the left that splits into the **left anterior descending**, or LAD, and the **circumflex**, and one on the right, the **right coronary artery**, or RCA. If the coronary arteries are blocked and unable to do their jobs, then the heart is left without oxygen and unable to do *its* job. Depriving the heart of oxygen for even a brief period of time will result in the death of some of the heart muscle—otherwise known as a heart attack.

The heart requires more oxygen when it's working hard, which is to say, when *you're* working hard. That's why many people with coronary artery disease classically experience chest pains when they're exerting themselves—jogging for instance, playing tennis, or even simply taking out the garbage. Your heart may be able to sustain itself at rest, but when you're exerting yourself, it needs more oxygen. The limited amount of oxygenated blood that reaches the cells through the diseased and partially blocked arteries simply isn't enough. These classic chest pains, also known as **angina,** are the diseased heart's signal that the coronary arteries aren't allowing enough oxygenated blood to reach the heart muscle.

When the amount of blood to a muscle is insufficient, that low-oxygen state is called **ischemia**. Coronary artery disease is often also called **ischemic heart disease** (IHD) as a result. A heart attack occurs when the coronary arteries are sufficiently blocked as to rob the heart muscle (the myocardium) of oxygen for long enough that part of the tissue dies (a condition called **infarction**). For this reason, a heart attack is called a **myocardial infarction,** or MI. **Peripheral artery disease,** or PAD, is when blockages occur in arteries other than the coronary arteries. These are no less serious: A stroke occurs when oxygen flow to the brain is blocked, and when oxygen flow to the limbs is blocked, the outcome can be gangrene.

ARTERIOSCLEROSIS: WHAT GOES WRONG

What prevents arteries from carrying oxygen-rich blood to the tissues they supply? **Arteriosclerosis** is the name for the process that results in what is commonly called "hardening of the arteries." A number of arterial disorders are grouped under this term. These disorders result in the narrowing and hardening of the arteries over time. One of the main steps in the **atherosclerosis** process is the deposit of fats in the inner walls of the arteries. These waxy deposits are called **plaque** and are made up of a combination of fats, cholesterol, cell waste products, proteins, and scarlike tissue. Obviously, a plaque deposit reduces the diameter of the inside of the artery, thereby reducing (or completely obstructing) blood flow. But early in the arteriosclerosis process, the diameter of the artery is *not* narrowed. Instead, the artery wall expands to accept the fatty deposits. In the early stages of the disease, the blood flow is totally normal. It's not until later in the disease process that the artery can no longer expand and the only place left for the fatty deposits to go is inward, blocking the blood flow. We used to think that gradual obstruction was the major cause of heart attacks, but we now know a little bit more about what happens during a stroke or a heart attack, and it's more complicated than a slowly clogging pipe.

Plaque Instability: The Real Culprit

Early plaque deposits start within the walls of the artery, creating a lesion. This is often the result of something irritating the blood vessel wall in a chronic way, followed by the artery's attempt to heal itself, which can result in a scarlike formation. These lesions sometimes rupture, causing blood to clot in the area. When that sudden blood clot occurs on top of a 50 percent blockage, it turns into a 100 percent blockage and results in a heart attack. It is only relatively recently that we learned that most heart attacks are caused by these 50 percent   blockages—not the 90 percenters we'd previously blamed. Certain kinds of plaque are more likely to rupture than others, so we're now much more interested in determining the causes of and treatments for this condition, which is called **plaque instability**.

Oxidation and inflammation are two common causes of plaque instability. Let's first look at oxidation.

Oxidation: Creating Toxic LDL

As you know, the human body simply cannot survive without oxygen. But this life-giving element can also have a corrosive effect on the cells in our body. Kitchen science provides the clearest example of the deleterious effects of oxygen: When you cut an apple and leave it out, the exposure to the oxygen in the air makes the flesh of the fruit turn brown. Cooks know that if you sprinkle the inside of the apple with some lemon juice, the fruit will stay white. The vitamin C in the lemon juice acts as an antioxidant—it protects the apple's cells from the oxygen in the air.

How does this work on the arterial level? Let's say you have the beginning of plaque starting in one of your arteries. As low-density lipoprotein (LDL), more popularly known as the "bad" cholesterol, is on its normal journey through the artery, it may be susceptible to oxidative damage either because of its chemical makeup or because of low antioxidant levels inside the LDL.

LDLs migrate into the artery wall; the smaller ones weasel their way in faster than the larger ones. Unfortunately, the smaller ones are more susceptible to oxidative damage. Once these LDLs get oxidized inside the artery wall, they become very attractive to the white blood cells whose job it is to clean up the area. If these white blood cells "clean up" too many oxidized LDLs, they die and release a chemical that makes the plaque unstable. It starts a very negative cycle: Since an injured artery is more likely to trap LDL, further injury to the artery is even more likely to occur. As the wall becomes more and more damaged, rupture and the accompanying heart attack are often the end result. In chapter 10, I'll discuss ways to help protect your arteries from this destructive cycle.

Inflammation: Swelling in the Arteries

Inflammation is another common cause of plaque instability. Inflammation is a natural process that occurs in an attempt to heal some damage or irritation.

White blood cells, the immune system's warriors, arrive at the scene of the crime to attack and eliminate infection. When you turn your ankle and it swells or your eye puffs up with conjunctivitis—even when an infected paper cut turns red and swells—that is inflammation.

White blood cells also rush to the rescue when the blood vessels of the heart are irritated by a high-fat meal or a hit of cigarette smoke. If the injury happens once, the body can heal itself in a few weeks. Unfortunately, when the injuries are chronic (a smoking habit, a chronically high-fat diet), the white blood cells can't keep up. They become obese and die. When this happens repeatedly, scarlike tissue forms in the shape of plaque. And inflammation also makes that plaque more likely to rupture. In other words, this form of atherosclerosis is a by-product of the body's effort to heal itself—when the injury is chronic and repetitive, the normal healing process becomes destructive.

As damaging as inflammation can be, it can also be a very useful diagnostic tool. When we see it, we know that there's a potential problem in the arteries. Now that we have the tests to measure it, we can use inflammation as an effective early warning sign of coronary artery disease.

Calcification: Arterial Lead Pipes

Another arterial disorder is **calcification,** or the presence of calcium in the walls of the blood vessel. As you may know, any cell in the body that contains DNA can activate certain genes and turn itself into another kind of cell (this is the theory behind stem cell research). When you have atherosclerosis for a long time, your body tries to repair the damage; one of the ways it does that is by turning the cells surrounding the arterial wall into a type of bone cell. When you have lesions containing calcium in the arterial walls, it's a clear sign of injury and repair—the hallmark of atherosclerosis. Eventually, the arteries can harden and appear a little like lead pipes.

Now this isn't necessarily a bad thing. In fact, this lead pipe effect can serve as protection. Soft plaques that haven't yet calcified can easily rupture and cause a heart attack, but the threat of rupture is lower once this process of calcification has been around for a while. Although some good can come of it, people with lots of calcium in their coronary arteries are at high risk of heart attack because their high calcium score indicates that they have many plaques. The more plaques you have, the more likely it is that one of them will rupture and cause a heart attack. Of course, you may have no signs of calcification and still have dangerous fatty buildup, so this isn't a foolproof sign. Nevertheless, any sign of calcification in a younger person is a reliable indicator of premature coronary heart disease.

Thrombosis: Blood Clots

Thrombosis is the blood's ability to clot, which prevents you from bleeding to death every time you cut yourself shaving.

Clotting is another way the body's natural healing mechanisms can be turned against it. Your blood is always clotting and unclotting in response to various stimuli, and that's fine, as long as there's a balance between the two. What you don't want is blood that has a marked tendency to clot—or an inability to unclot.

Here's why clotting is a problem. Imagine that you have some unstable plaque causing a partial blockage in your artery. When that plaque ruptures like a volcano, it releases toxic chemicals, which can stimulate the formation of a clot over the ruptured blockage. Sometimes that clot is big enough to block the artery itself, and sometimes it breaks loose and drifts downstream where it backs up behind another partial blockage and closes off the artery.

Another clotting problem can happen before your arteriosclerosis is even very advanced. Let's say that you have a small amount of damage to the artery, and you do something—say, smoke a cigarette or have a really fatty meal—that irritates the injury. The body rushes to heal the injury; a clot forms and eventually turns into a scar. Then you have another fatty meal, or another cigarette, or a routine infection, and the same thing happens all over again. That scar tissue builds up and will eventually become a blockage.

Platelets are a big culprit in this tendency to clot. They do this in a number of ways. Either they get "sticky" and bunch up, attaching themselves to the side of the artery, or they release chemicals that make blood clotting more likely. You've probably heard about the connection between aspirin and heart health, and you may even be taking a baby aspirin every day on your doctor's recommendation. Aspirin mildly poisons platelets, which makes your blood less likely to clot.

Certain of the metabolic traits that we'll be discussing later in the book increase your tendency to clot. We call anything that makes blood likely to clot **thrombogenic,** and as you'll see throughout the book, we'll be steering you in the direction of things that make your blood less sticky.

Vasoreactivity: Arterial Spasm

Another concept that's been drawing lots of attention lately is a relatively new discovery, called vasoreactivity. This is basically equivalent to a muscle spasm, but one that affects the arteries. Cardiologists are paying close attention to this emerging research because vasoreactivity appears to be a reliable indicator of the overall health of the arteries.

There's a kind of muscular corkscrew around the outside of each artery, which helps it to expand and contract in the course of its normal physiological process. Think of a hose. If the walls of the hose are too soft, the flow of liquid will be hard to control. But if the walls are firmer, the flow of the liquid is more easily directed. This muscular corkscrew on the outside of the arterial walls tightens to make the arteries more firm, so that the blood flow within is more easily directed and managed. When you stand up after lying down for a long time, your arteries constrict slightly to keep blood flow moving to your brain. The lightheadedness you feel sometimes when you get up too quickly gives you an idea of what life would be like if your arteries didn't have this normal vasoreactivity.

But too much vasoreactivity can be a problem, especially in someone with existing coronary heart disease. You don't want your arteries to seize suddenly, especially not on top of a lesion that's already causing a 50 percent blockage. If your artery clamps down too much, it'll stop blood flow through the vessel entirely, and that can result in a heart attack. So this combination of abnormal constriction and partial blockages is particularly dangerous. If we can encourage the arteries to be more relaxed, then we can improve the amount of blood going to all parts of the heart and even help prevent arteries from clamping down abnormally. The size of the blockage may not have changed, but by preventing artery spasm, we can prevent a sudden relative increase in the percentage of the artery that's blocked. Think of it this way: Let's say you have a 50 percent blockage in an artery with a 1-inch diameter, so the blockage is ½ inch. When the artery spasms, the already reduced diameter gets even smaller so now the 50 percent blockage becomes 100 percent.

As you'll see, I address this concept of vasoreactivity in various places throughout the book. You'll learn about things that can cause an unfavorable increase in **vasoconstriction**, or the tendency of the arteries to clamp down suddenly, such as diets rich in saturated fats, smoking, low high-density lipoprotein (HDL), high triglycerides and LDL cholesterol, and cocaine, just to name a few. As we'll later discuss, certain metabolic imbalances can also increase vasoconstriction. Factors that help promote vasorelaxation, which can be very helpful in counteracting this tendency, include fish oils, diets rich in soy, and exercise.

If you're facing this particular issue, you'll learn about all the ways you can fight back—from treating the metabolic imbalance that gives rise to this problem (in chapter 4) to getting on the specific diet and exercise programs that will help neutralize it (in chapters 7 and 8).

I hope this provides you with a basic understanding of the rudimentary workings of a healthy heart and of one that's broken. The traditional view of coronary artery disease has been along the lines of a stopped-up drainpipe, but you can now appreciate that the processes that give rise to coronary artery disease are far more dynamic and complex than a simple blockage. The more precise we can be in targeting and isolating the particular ways that these processes interact to compromise your heart health, the better equipped we are to launch an effective counteroffensive.

You're now ready to construct your own Cardiac Fingerprint, a process that will lead you to a better understanding of the state of your own heart.

2

THE CARDIAC FINGERPRINT: A COMPREHENSIVE RISK ASSESSMENT

BUILDING YOUR CARDIAC FINGERPRINT is the first step in our journey toward a new paradigm in cardiac prevention and care. At the end of that journey, you'll have a number of custom-made Prescriptions to share with your physician, designed to help you outwit your cardiac destiny. But you can't find a solution to a problem you don't know you have, so the first step we must take is to conduct a candid assessment of the person under consideration: *you*.

We'll be calling the results of this comprehensive assessment your Cardiac Fingerprint. Like a fingerprint, it will be uniquely yours. As we move away from the one-size-fits-all school of thought on cardiac care, we need instead to focus on what makes each cardiac profile unique. And in order to truly understand how your specific cardiovascular system may be attacked, we need to know not only all the variables that go into your particular cardiac makeup, but also how those variables work together. Like a fingerprint, which is really an intricate combination of swirls, lines, and loops working together to create a unique and defining pattern, your unique cardiac identity will be found in the complex interplay among otherwise discrete factors.

Your Cardiac Fingerprint will bring together many disparate pieces of information about you: your personal medical history, your family's medical history, your environment, your lifestyle choices, the composition of your blood, and eventually, your genetic code. This will be a much more sophisticated and detailed assessment than the ones previously available. Much of the material that you encounter in this assessment process will be new to you, but I think you'll find that even answers to questions you've answered a thousand times before will look different when viewed through the lens of your cardiac profile as a whole. It is only when we look at the entire weave of factors, together and apart, that we can begin to put together a true accounting of the risks you face.

Like a fingerprint, there are elements in your Cardiac Fingerprint that cannot be changed. A predisposition toward coronary heart disease may be genetically determined, for example, and you cannot change your genes. Other factors that impact your risk are also fixed, like your age: A certain degree of normal wear and tear occurs naturally over time, so your risk rises proportionately as your age increases. There are other fixed factors that lie beyond your control as well.

But here's how that complex interplay of factors actually works to our advantage. You can't control some things, but that doesn't mean you're totally out of the driver's seat.

> **No matter how hard-wired coronary heart disease is in your genes, the outcome isn't determined! Your ability to control your lifestyle choices gives you a great deal of authority over the condition of your arteries and heart.**

Thankfully, the incontrovertible aspects of your Cardiac Fingerprint, like your genes and your age, aren't the only things determining whether or not you'll get coronary heart disease. In fact, there is no one root cause of coronary artery disease: It comes about as a result of this interaction between your genes, your physical condition, your inherited predispositions, and your lifestyle. So the fact that the process is dynamic is good news. It means that no matter what fixed negatives there might be in your Cardiac Fingerprint, if you can keep the host of other gears in that apparatus well-oiled and in good working order, then you can override the destiny encoded in your genes.

If there's one concept that I'd like you to take away from this book, it's this: Since you *can* control so many of the environmental and lifestyle issues that contribute to the onset and the progression of coronary heart disease, you also have the power to cut coronary heart disease off at the pass. By itself, a genetic predisposition toward coronary heart disease would seal your fate, making this disease impossible to defeat. But the fact that these fixed genetic factors can be affected by a myriad of other things that you *can* control means that you have the power to alter your own cardiac future.

CORONARY HEART DISEASE IS PREVENTABLE AND TREATABLE

As you'll see in part 2, the Prescription section of the book, there's a surprising amount you can do to prevent, treat, and even reverse coronary heart disease. Moreover, truly incredible results can often be achieved just by making sensible lifestyle changes like quitting smoking and losing weight—with medications added when necessary. In short, once we've determined what the most appropriate programs are for your cardiac profile, chances are very good that you can turn this disease around.

It may also surprise you to learn that lifestyle factors aren't the only things that are under your control. You can also influence many of the inherited factors that affect your risk of coronary heart disease. Yes, you're stuck with the genes you were born with, and it's certainly true that many conditions that have a degenerative effect on the arteries, such as elevated triglycerides, insulin resistance, and high blood pressure, are to some extent genetically determined. But you nonetheless have much influence over these conditions. By controlling your weight, getting on diet and exercise programs that have been customized to your cardiac profile, and when necessary, taking medications that take into account your complete metabolic profile, you can dramatically reduce the danger you face.

In fact, our sphere of influence runs even deeper than that. As you'll see, with the right plans in place, we're able to change your very physiology—the way your body works at a metabolic level. You can turn some of these genes on and off! For example, we can change the particle size of the lipoproteins your body produces, thereby altering a significant danger. And that's as close as you can come to outsmarting your own genes. How's that for taking charge of your own cardiac destiny?

In the second half of this book, we'll give you and your doctor the tools to help you make those changes in the most constructive, efficient, and effective ways possible. So while you may have inherited a predisposition for coronary heart disease along with that antique grandfather clock, your genes don't necessarily mean that you'll fall victim to it. The way you live and the treatment you seek directly affect your heart health—it's that *combination* of inherited and lifestyle risks that puts you in the danger zone. Even if you're one of the unlucky people who inherited a host of risk factors, you're not condemned to relentlessly progressive coronary heart disease. In most cases, once you know that you're at risk, the lifestyle and medication choices you make can either delay the onset of the disease indefinitely or slow its progression so that you can still live a heart-healthy life.

"BUT . . . "

There's only one "but." In order to make an effective preemptive strike against coronary heart disease, *you have to know that you're at risk, and you need to know precisely what factors are putting you in harm's way.*

That's why we need a much more advanced system of assessment than the one we've been using. A quick family history and a cholesterol test simply won't tell us what we need to know to put you back in the driver's seat. We need to determine just how much danger you're in and how aggressive your counteroffensive must be. And to do that, we need in-depth assessment tools that will detail your metabolic, genetic, and lifestyle picture. We need all of the information contained in the Cardiac Fingerprint. This is why assessing your risk is an essential first step in beating coronary heart disease.

THE FIRST STEP: KNOW THAT YOU'RE AT RISK

All of our customized diets, personalized exercise programs, and powerful medications are helpless in the face of ignorance.

Remember all those stealth heart attack victims we talked about earlier? Those people in "perfect" health, struck down suddenly by massive heart attacks that no one, not even their doctors, saw coming? In truth, those heart attacks were caused by a simple lack of information. Since those people didn't know they were at risk, they weren't able to avail themselves of the weapons at their disposal to remedy their problem. Now that we have the diagnostic tools to determine who's at risk—and precisely how much risk they face—there's simply no excuse for getting blindsided in this way.

By finding out your risk level, you can take charge of your fate. If your Personal Risk Profile indicates even a moderate level of risk, you'll want to consider also getting more advanced screening tests that will reveal any underlying metabolic imbalances that might signal additional cardiac risk. If your Personal Risk Profile indicates a high or extreme level of risk, you'll definitely want to proceed with those tests—they might save your life!

TREATMENT: HOW AGGRESSIVE SHOULD WE BE?

Your Cardiac Fingerprint not only indicates where to focus your energies but will also help you to gauge the level of force necessary in your counteroffensive. If the risks are severe, you and your physician know to attack aggressively; if your risk profile is lower, you can afford to take a more long-term approach.

In other words, your complete risk profile enables your physician to treat *you* specifically and personally: It is the cornerstone of this new, individualized, patient-specific brand of medicine.

Let's look at two examples: The following two patients came in to see me. Richard is a man in his fifties, diabetic, and 30 pounds overweight. He's in a stressful line of work, he considers the walk from the office to his car "exercise," and he lost his father and his older brother to heart attacks early in their lives. Jane is a moderately fit, premenopausal woman with no family history of coronary heart disease.

Even if these two people have *exactly* the same cholesterol numbers, I would treat them differently and recommend very different sorts of interventions.

As far as I'm concerned, Richard is a ticking time bomb. I want to get all the information I possibly can about the specifics of his genetic predisposition toward coronary heart disease. When I have that information, I'm going to go after his disease (or predisease condition, if he's lucky) aggressively, with medication and conscientious lifestyle changes.

We're going to treat Jane a little differently. Although we certainly will work to see an improvement in her numbers, we can generally spend more time encouraging her to change her way of life before placing her on medication. By virtue of her gender, her genes, and her lifestyle, she runs a lower risk of experiencing a cardiac event.

Risk is relative, which is why treatment must focus on the particular patient, not just on the numbers. Let's push the example a little further. We do a series of advanced tests on Jane and Richard, and in both cases, we discover a risk factor that multiplies their risk by 300 percent. The cookie-cutter approach would have us treat them the same way, since their scores are the same. But Jane's risk of heart attack before the tests was 1 percent in the next 5 years, so although that risk factor trebles her risk, her ultimate risk is only 3 percent in the next 5 years. While important, that's still a relatively low number, certainly nothing that requires immediate medication.

Richard, on the other hand, isn't so lucky. His lifestyle, physical condition, and family history made his risk of experiencing a heart attack about 30 percent in the next 5 years before the additional screening tests. Now we know his risk is tripled, which leaves him with a staggering 90 percent chance of cardiac event. There's no time to waste—we have to do everything within our power to get this guy out of danger.

This is why a numbers-only approach to coronary heart disease can be misleading: We need to have a full picture of all the risk factors before we can determine how aggressively to pursue treatment. These two people have the same cholesterol numbers and the same metabolic disorder—but informed treatment decisions are virtually impossible unless we take their *complete* risk profiles into account.

KNOW THINE ENEMY: WHICH RISK FACTORS ARE PUTTING *YOU* IN HARM'S WAY?

Another reason that it's so important to establish your risk profile: You can't know what to fix until you know precisely what factors are putting you at risk.

Let's go back to Richard from the example above. His total cholesterol is 190 mg/dl, so those numbers alone are not all that worrisome. It's only when those numbers are placed in the context of all the other factors that we begin to see just how high his level of risk is. It's true that the genetic dice are loaded against him because his family history, one of the strongest risk predictors, is so bad. If coronary heart disease was exclusively determined by genetics, my advice to Richard would be to buy life insurance. But, as we know, lifestyle changes can commute the premature death sentence passed on Richard by his genes.

His unhealthy choices—his stress patterns, the facts that he's overweight and doesn't exercise—all exacerbate the conditions he inherited. You might remember the ad for Clairol hair color, "Why not change the things you can?" It's a good question: Why not address those risk factors in your Cardiac Fingerprint that are under your control?

Richard doesn't know how much of a difference cleaning up his lifestyle would make. And it's possible that he simply wasn't motivated to make lifestyle improvements before he discovered that he was at a 90 percent risk of heart attack. Now that he's got his Cardiac Fingerprint, he knows what his risk factors are and which ones he can change. His overall risk profile results might be scary, but they're still an advance warning. If Richard chooses to see the writing on the wall, these results could save his life.

Learning about the risk factors contributing to his cardiac threat puts Richard back in control. Nothing is going to give him better genes, but he can certainly lose weight, adopt the correct diet for his heart profile, and start exercising—and those things will appreciably decrease the intensity of his risk. He doesn't need to change his genes; he just needs to impact the gene-lifestyle dynamic to find a healthier balance between the two.

I hope this has convinced you of the importance of taking the self-assessment test. So let's get to it!

In the next chapter, I'll walk you through the particular risk factors that appear in the Personal Risk Profile. I think it's helpful and necessary to familiarize you with each of the components contributing to your risk level before simply giving you a score. But if you feel you really can't wait, go ahead and flip ahead to the test, and then return to the early part of the chapter for a fuller explanation of what each entry in the test really means.

3

THE FACTORS PUTTING
YOU AT RISK

YOUR PERSONAL RISK PROFILE is the first entry in your Cardiac Fingerprint. It is a unique self-assessment tool designed to calibrate your level of risk. Composed of simple questions that don't require any lab work, it can be completed without a doctor's help. This will help you and your doctor determine just how vigilant you need to be, and whether or not you should consider further testing. Please note: This *isn't* a diagnostic test. In other words, the results of this test do not give us any diagnostic information about the current risk status of your heart and cardiovascular system. (That comes later, with the Advanced Metabolic Marker Profile.) What this self-assessment test does offer is a reliable indication of whether you are at risk for the underlying disorders that cause coronary heart disease or a cardiac event—and if so, how far out you're standing on that risk axis.

WHAT ARE THESE RISK FACTORS?

You hear the term *risk factor* everywhere these days, and we'll be using it a lot throughout this book as well. The self-assessment test that you're about to take is designed to analyze your particular combination of risk factors for coronary heart disease or cardiac event. In the next few pages, we'll take a closer look at what these risk factors are, how they impact your heart and health, and why these are the ones flagged when we're evaluating coronary heart disease risk.

The risk factors I'm concerned with can be grouped into five basic categories.

    I. **Fixed factors:** Things that you do not have the power to change, such as your age and gender

    II. **Inherited factors:** Your family history, especially as it relates to your heart

    III. **Medical factors:** Medical conditions that affect heart health

    IV. **Physical factors:** Physical traits that act as predictors of cardiac danger

    V. **Lifestyle factors:** Behaviors and habits that affect your heart health, such as smoking, diet, exercise, stress patterns, and so on

I. Fixed Factors: The Things You Cannot Change

Some of the factors that affect your risk for coronary heart disease—gender, age, and ethnicity—are beyond your control. But as you'll see, in many cases, you can change the degree of their negative impact on your heart.

- Gender
- Age
- Ethnicity

How does gender affect your risk for coronary heart disease?

Simply put, men are at higher risk for coronary heart disease than women. Or, to be more precise, men are at higher risk for heart disease than *premenopausal* women.

What's the explanation for this gender gap? Women's bodies afford a certain degree of natural protection against coronary heart disease by producing female hormones such as estrogen. Unfortunately, the heart-preserving benefits of estrogen last only as long as the body is actively producing it at peak levels. So a woman's risk of coronary heart disease rises significantly once she goes through menopause. One of the strongest arguments for hormone therapy (HT) is that replaced estrogen may protect against coronary heart disease. However, HT is currently controversial. For more information regarding menopause, HT, and heart disease, please see chapter 9, where we review the pros and cons in more detail.

While the protective benefits of estrogen are wonderful, I am troubled by the fact that women have been left out of the coronary heart disease equation. By now, we know that women must take coronary heart disease just as seriously as men must. This isn't a man's disease, and any message that indicates otherwise is not only false, but dangerous. I'd like to take this opportunity to remind you that heart disease—not breast cancer—is the leading killer of American women. So women can't afford to be any less vigilant than men when it comes to their heart health.

What toll does your age take on your heart?

We take it pretty much for granted that our body parts will eventually wear out as we get old. But experts working on longevity genetics at the Human Genome Project estimate that were it not for intervening issues, humans should be able to live about 150 years. What that tells us is that it isn't normal wear and tear that's wearing out our bodies prematurely, but chronic disease. And one of those chronic diseases is atherosclerosis.

You can't turn back the hands of time when it comes to aging; the clock keeps ticking. But the simple progression of years does not in itself explain coronary heart disease. The risk of heart disease absolutely does increase with age, but that's because the longer we live, the longer our bodies are being exposed to chronic **atherogenic** conditions—the conditions that cause coronary artery disease. The more years we spend on this planet, the more high-fat meals we're likely to eat, for instance, and the more secondhand smoke we're likely to inhale. And the greater the atherogenic burden that is placed on your body, the faster you'll wear out your cardiovascular system. So aging isn't just how many years you've racked up, but what you *do*—both to and for your body—in those years.

Although you can't lower your chronological age, you can determine the "age" of your arteries by keeping them in good condition and in that way directly influence whether that first heart attack happens at 45 or 85.

How does your ethnicity affect your risk?

It may not be politically correct, but it's true: Certain ethnic groups are at higher risk for coronary heart disease. In some cases, your ethnicity can increase your risk to an even greater extent than high cholesterol numbers or smoking. Asian Indians, Native Americans, Mexican-Americans, and those of Native Hawaiian or Pacific Islander descent appear to be at a particularly high risk.

This ethnicity issue is a good example of the dynamic between your genes and environment and of the importance of making that balance work to your greatest advantage. People belonging to these populations are at special and increased risk *if* they allow themselves to become overweight. So don't waste time blaming your ancestry—just make sure you're keeping trim!

Like all these fixed factors, knowing that you're at higher risk simply by virtue of your ethnic background can be incredibly valuable. It enables you to get the upper hand by eliminating all the risk factors that you *can*.

II. Your Genes: It's a Family Affair

The conditions that give rise to coronary heart disease are largely inherited. As you'll see when you take the self-assessment test, having heart disease close to home is a real sign of risk, so when I find out that one of my patients has a first-degree relative with coronary heart disease, it immediately sends up a red flag.

- A first-degree relative with coronary heart disease

Do you have a family history of coronary heart disease?

The genetic conditions that cause heart disease tend to pass from generation to generation in what we call a **Mendelian dominant inheritance pattern.** Translation: A parent has a 50 percent chance of passing these genetic conditions along to offspring. And that means that each child has a 50 percent chance of getting it—not that one kid will and one kid won't. Both may, or both may not, but they each have an equal chance of inheriting a trait that dramatically increases their coronary heart disease risk. A first-degree relative (father, mother, sibling) with heart disease is one of the strongest indications that you may be at risk.

When I see patients for the first time, I always ask them to construct their own coronary heart disease family pedigree. Although this is one of the line items in the following questionnaire, I think that actually seeing a visual representation of your family's history in one place—the intersection between cardiology and genealogy—can be worthwhile. I recommend that you take a moment to do this exercise along with me.

Here's how you make a family pedigree.

First, draw your family tree. Here's a sample.

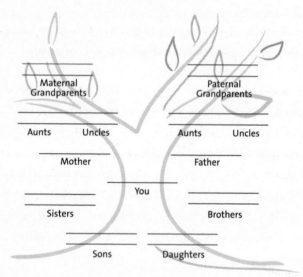

Obviously, if your mother has nine brothers and your father is an only child, your chart will look a little different. All you need to do is to make a list of your primary relatives: grandparents, parents, siblings, and your children.

Now go through the family tree you've created and place a heart above everyone who you know had coronary heart disease or suffered a heart attack. If you have additional information about their condition (like whether anyone had a history of high cholesterol or the age at which they first experienced the disease), include those details as well.

Add a square (to represent a sugar cube) next to each individual you know had, or currently suffers from, diabetes. Diabetes, as you'll see, is another hereditary condition that can often be forestalled or even prevented through lifestyle. And developing diabetes (or a prediabetic condition) formidably raises coronary heart disease risk.

Now sit back and look at your handiwork. You can probably draw your own conclusions from the evidence in front of you. If your granny died of heart failure at 96, and she's the only heart on your profile, then although you do have a history of coronary heart disease, we can safely say that your genes are on your side. On the other hand, if your dad's three brothers were all victims of heart attacks before 45, then that's a pretty good indication that you're in a dangerous situation.

But even if your sheet is covered with hearts and sugar cubes, don't let that discourage you. Remember, your genes are not your destiny: Lifestyle comes to the rescue! Let's say your brother has type 2 diabetes. That puts you at higher risk, both for developing diabetes and for coronary heart disease. But your brother has also been 70 pounds overweight since he was 14 years old. If you work hard to stay in decent shape by eating properly, exercising, and managing your weight and lipids, you're already doing something significant to manage that genetic risk. And we can test you for other underlying conditions that you can also treat in order to take your prevention efforts to the next level.

III. Physical Factors: Mirror, Mirror, on the Wall

Certain physical traits, oddly enough, are predictors of heart attack risk. There's nothing you can do about them, but if you have them, that's added motivation for you to make sure you're taking action in your lifestyle to minimize risk where you can.

- Arcus senilis
- Coronary ear crease
- Vertex male-pattern baldness

What's arcus senilis?

Look at your eye. There's a black dot in the center, which is the pupil, and a colored part around that dot, which is the iris. If there is a thin, yellow-white line encircling the pupil and separating those two areas, you're at higher risk for coronary heart disease. (The line may be slightly disconnected, so that there's an arc on the bottom and an arc at the top, but it still counts.)

That creamy line, called **arcus senilis**, is a cholesterol deposit, and it almost always indicates a very high level of LDL blood cholesterol. We see this most often in the elderly, but it's not infrequent in younger people, and it is a significant indicator that you're in danger of coronary heart disease.

What's a coronary ear crease, and how do you know if you have it?

Look for a 45-degree crease, running from back to front (pointing toward your eyebrow) in *both* earlobes.

Here's a terrific example of the way a vigilant, observant physician can make a real breakthrough discovery just by paying close attention to his patients. A cardiologist in Sweden happened to notice that a substantial number of his heart attack patients had a certain kind of crease in their earlobes. He got some money together to look into it, and lo and behold: They discovered that there was a correlation between this kind of ear crease and an increased rate of coronary heart disease.

Obviously, this ear crease isn't causing myocardial infarctions. Since both heart disease and ear creases are inherited, we think that these genes are somehow bundled together. As crazy as it sounds, this ear crease does act as an informal predictive marker for increased risk. And the creases must be on *both* sides—researchers determined that a crease on one side had less to do with heart attack risk than with which side the patient favored in bed!

What's vertex male-pattern baldness, and how do you know if you have it?

Here's one more thing to worry about: How you lose your hair may affect your risk for angina, nonfatal heart attacks, and the need for bypass surgery.

A number of studies have shown that men who are thinning on top are at higher risk for coronary heart disease. If you have vertex baldness, meaning that you're bald on the top of your head and down the center, with hair on the sides like Bozo the Clown, your risk is substantially higher than in men who have all their hair or even in men with receding hairlines or baldness at the front. All clowning aside, this vertex male-pattern style of balding is a real predictor and something to take seriously.

It's not clear why there's a link. It might be connected to the higher rates of testosterone associated with bald men (this might also be the basis for the old wives' tale that bald men are more virile). Or the male-pattern baldness gene might be packaged with a gene that causes coronary heart disease, so that they show up together.

Again, since there's nothing you can do about these physical predictors (hair plugs don't count!), if you have them, you'll want to marshal your energies toward controlling those risk factors that you can.

IV. Medical Factors: The Leg Bone's Connected to the Hipbone

Our physiological systems do not exist in a vacuum. The human body wrote the book on synergy; it's a precisely calibrated, interconnected, and interdependent system. So when one part of your body has a problem, chances are good that at least one other part of the body will (eventually) suffer as well. The heart is no exception: It is keenly affected by a number of physical conditions that afflict other parts of the body.

You might be thinking that if you have one or more of these medical conditions, the horse is already out of the barn. It's not true. Of course, you should do everything within your power to prevent these illnesses, but if you already have them, you should know that careful management of these conditions can help to prevent the damage they do to your heart.

- Diabetes
- High blood pressure
- Peripheral artery disease
- Chronic infections

Are you diabetic?

If you have diabetes or there's diabetes in your family, you're at considerably higher risk for coronary heart disease. In fact, heart disease is the number-one cause of diabetes-related death, and adults with diabetes are two to four times as likely to die of cardiovascular disease as adults without diabetes are.

Insulin is the hormone that regulates your blood sugar. After you eat, your pancreas releases insulin so that your blood sugar doesn't spike and drop dramatically according to your food intake. People with diabetes are either unable to manufacture enough insulin (the relatively rare type 1), or their cells have become resistant to its effects (the more common type 2). People with diabetes have to monitor and help to regulate their own insulin and blood sugar levels, since their bodies are incapable of doing it.

If you have a family history of diabetes, you must do everything within your power to ensure that this condition doesn't manifest itself in you. That includes following a healthy diet, exercising regularly, and maintaining an appropriate weight.

If you're already diabetic or insulin resistant, controlling your blood sugar levels is essential. Insulin itself is atherogenic, and high levels of it in the bloodstream irritate the heart. Chronically high blood sugar has been linked to low HDL ("good") cholesterol, high triglyceride levels, high blood pressure, and arterial hardening—all things that can increase your risk.

When you take good care of your blood sugar, you're taking good care of your heart.

Do you have high blood pressure?

It's estimated that one out of every four Americans suffers from high blood pressure. That's too many people!

High blood pressure can cause blurred vision and blindness and reduce kidney function, which means the kidneys are less efficient at removing waste from the bloodstream. High blood pressure makes the heart work harder than it needs to and is directly linked to coronary heart disease and stroke, the first and third leading causes of death in America. It's also statistically linked to LDL pattern B, one of the more serious metabolic issues that I'll be discussing in this book.

Mildly elevated blood pressure can often be controlled through lifestyle measures such as diet and exercise. Why wait until you're in a danger zone to combat the problem with medication? And why settle for the blood pressure of a highly stressed stockbroker when you can have the blood pressure of a marathon runner?

While we're on the topic of elevated blood pressure, let's take a minute to discuss a theme that you'll be hearing from me a lot. I am not a big fan of "cutoff numbers"—the idea that there's a numerical line in the sand where danger starts. I understand why cutoff numbers are necessary, but the drawbacks are just as real. With blood pressure, I can show you a good example of why we have to be careful when we apply standardized cutoff numbers.

The idea that a blood pressure of 130 is dangerous but that you're okay at 129 is absurd. As far as I'm concerned, it represents the worst aspect of this cookie-cutter approach to medicine. We have to get away from this slavery to the numbers if we're going to beat this disease: Each person must have *his or her own* best numbers as a target goal. If you're at risk for other reasons, and your blood pressure is on the high side even if it's not putting you in the danger zone, then in my opinion, you still need to bring it down.

Do you have peripheral artery disease?

You'd be surprised how often people fail to make the connection between atherosclerosis in other sites in the body and atherosclerosis in the heart.

If you have a history of blocked arteries in places other than the heart, such as your legs, neck, or abdomen, then you're also at an increased risk for coronary artery disease.

Do you have chronic and/or frequent infections?

Recent studies have linked coronary heart disease risk to total pathogen load—in other words, the more infections you have, the more likely you are to develop heart disease.

Why would a garden-variety infection like gum disease or bronchitis have anything to do with your heart? We think this is linked to the arterial inflammation issue. Even a regular bronchial infection may cause some damage, and when the body goes to heal that infection, it actually makes the problem worse by creating scar tissue that can turn into arterial plaque.

So if you have serious colds, bronchitis, pneumonia, ear infections, urinary tract infections, or gum inflammation more than twice a year or chronic gingivitis, you may be at increased risk. Keep your immune system in fighting shape and treat infections properly—you'll have a better winter, and it's a good thing to do for your heart.

V. Lifestyle Factors: Why Not Change the Things You *Can*?

Almost all of the risk factors we've discussed so far can be influenced, if not completely neutralized, through lifestyle. How you cope with the risk factors that *are* in your control can mean the difference between life and death. Let's take a look at the lifestyle choices that can make such a powerful difference in your cardiac destiny.

Obviously, everyone should be vigilant about maintaining a heart-healthy lifestyle, no matter what your risk profile looks like. This is especially important for those of you who have gotten a heads-up that you're at high risk— whether it's because you're older, because you have a family history of coronary heart disease, or because you're balding like Bozo. This is your chance to take matters into your own hands and improve your odds.

- Smoking
- Weight control
- Exercise
- Stress

Do you smoke cigarettes?

If you're a smoker in this day and age, then I'm sure I'm not going to be the first person to give you a lecture about it. I will say this: It's killing you.

You probably know all the horrifying statistics about lung cancer and emphysema, but many people don't realize just how bad smoking is for their arteries. Did you know that coronary heart disease kills more smokers than cancer does? It's true.

Smoking lowers HDL and HDL2b, the "good" kinds of cholesterol, and it lowers one of the body's natural antioxidants, a protective natural enzyme called **paraoxanase**. The toxic agents in tobacco literally poison the cells in the walls of the arteries, making them more susceptible to plaque and to rupture. Cigarette smoke causes already damaged arteries to constrict in an unhealthy way, which puts you at risk for sudden heart attack and contributes to the tendency of the blood to clot, which increases your risk of peripheral artery disease, coronary artery disease, heart attack, and stroke. In short, it couldn't be worse.

But you can turn it around, just like that. Someone who quits smoking has only half of a smoker's risk of coronary artery disease—no matter how long they smoked before quitting. And after 5 years, your risk has dropped considerably.

A great many of my patients and friends are former smokers, and I know how very difficult it can be to give up this habit. There's no magic formula. You have to decide you're going to stop, and then you have to just do it. There are things that can help you to quit, from nicotine gum to the patch to medication to hypnotism, and I can't recommend one method over another; everyone has to find the form of support that works best for them. Whether you choose to use an aid or go cold turkey, I strongly recommend that you do whatever you have to do in order to quit.

Do you live or work with a smoker?

People who are in constant contact with secondhand smoke may be at as much risk as those who smoke cigarettes themselves.

More and more cities are outlawing cigarette smoking in their restaurants and bars, and it's already illegal to smoke in the workplace, but there are still holdouts. You have every right to ask the smoker in your life to take it outside: They're choosing to injure themselves, but their unhealthy decision has a direct consequence on your health. And you may be doing them a favor: Shivering on the porch every time they have a craving may give them the incentive to quit.

Are you overweight?

Obesity is one of the most pressing health issues in America, primarily because it affects so many of the body's other systems.

We'll talk about the effects of weight on heart health at much greater length in the segment of the book on weight control. But suffice it to say that carrying extra weight is one of the worst things you can do for your body. When you're overweight, you're carrying pounds of inactive tissue. Being overweight strains your joints, your back, and your neck and interferes with the way your essential body processes work, especially your heart and cardiovascular system.

If my patients leave my office with one take-away, it's this: Lose the extra weight you're carrying, and I will guarantee an improvement in your numbers and overall heart health. I have literally *hundreds* of stories about people who were able to completely change their cardiac risk profile simply by losing weight.

The body mass index (BMI) is a good way to tell if you're carrying too much weight for your frame (see the table on page 34). All you have to know is how tall you are and how much you weigh.

According to the National Institutes of Health, a BMI of less than 18.5 means that you're underweight. You're healthy from 18.5 to 24.9, overweight from 25 to 29.9, and obese over 30.

So that gives you a baseline. But there's more: A study published in the *New England Journal of Medicine* has shown that men with BMIs over 26.5 and women with BMIs over 25 are at a much higher risk for cardiac event.

Many people feel overwhelmed by the idea of controlling their weight, but I believe it contains one of the most empowering concepts out there: You can beat one of the most significant factors contributing to coronary heart disease simply by controlling what you put into your mouth! We'll explore this very simple yet powerful notion at much greater length in part 2.

What's your waist circumference?

Waist circumference is another blunt tool we use to judge overweight.

One problem with BMI is that it doesn't take into account the very significant difference between muscle and fat mass. A 140-pound woman who exercises regularly may have a significant amount of very heavy muscle, which will result in a higher BMI although she's not really fat but in very good physical condition. When BMI is used in concert with waist circumference, we have a little more information.

Where people carry the added weight affects their risk for coronary heart disease. Some people gain weight in their thighs and rear end, which gives them a pear shape; some people get a big stomach, which makes them look more like an apple. Those people who carry their weight in their abdomen are the ones at greater risk for coronary heart disease.

To determine your waist circumference, take a tape measure and measure snugly around your waist. If your waist circumference exceeds the guidelines below, you're considered to be overweight and at higher risk for heart disease.

Men: more than 40 inches (or 102 centimeters)
Women: more than 35 inches (or 88 centimeters)

Do you exercise?

Like diet, exercise is one of the most significant lifestyle factors that can prevent coronary heart disease. In fact, there is even some evidence that vigorous regular exercise can roll existing heart disease back. Exercise can put you on the road to a cure!

But in order to reap the benefits of exercise, you have to do it vigorously and regularly. You have to exercise for a good amount of time each time you do it, and you have to sustain a regular routine or pattern of exercise over

(continued on page 36)

CALCULATE YOUR BODY MASS INDEX

To find your body mass index (BMI), locate your height in the left column. Move across the chart (to the right) until you hit your approximate weight. Then follow that column down to the corresponding BMI number at the bottom of the chart.

Height (in.)								
58	91	96	100	105	110	115	119	124
59	94	99	104	109	114	119	124	128
60	97	102	107	112	118	123	128	133
61	100	106	111	116	122	127	132	137
62	104	109	115	120	126	131	136	142
63	107	113	118	124	130	135	141	146
64	110	116	122	128	134	140	145	151
65	114	120	126	132	138	144	150	156
66	118	124	130	136	142	148	155	161
67	121	127	134	140	146	153	159	166
68	125	131	138	144	151	158	164	171
69	128	135	142	149	155	162	169	176
70	132	139	146	153	160	167	174	181
71	136	143	150	157	165	172	179	186
72	140	147	154	162	169	177	184	191
73	144	151	159	166	174	182	189	197
74	148	155	163	171	179	186	194	202
75	152	160	168	176	184	192	200	208
76	156	164	172	180	189	197	205	213
BMI	19	20	21	22	23	24	25	26

Body Weight (lb.)

129	134	138	143	148	153	158	162	167
133	138	143	148	153	158	163	168	173
138	143	148	153	158	163	168	174	179
143	148	153	158	164	169	174	180	185
147	153	158	164	169	175	180	186	191
152	158	163	169	175	180	186	191	197
157	163	169	174	180	186	192	197	204
162	168	174	180	186	192	198	204	210
167	173	179	186	192	198	204	210	216
172	178	185	191	198	204	211	217	223
177	184	190	197	203	210	216	223	230
182	189	196	203	209	216	223	230	236
188	195	202	209	216	222	229	236	243
193	200	208	215	222	229	236	243	250
199	206	213	221	228	235	242	250	258
204	212	219	227	235	242	250	257	265
210	218	225	233	241	249	256	264	272
216	224	232	240	248	256	264	272	279
221	230	238	246	254	263	271	279	287
27	**28**	**29**	**30**	**31**	**32**	**33**	**34**	**35**

many years to gain the optimal results. That's why you want to adopt a routine that suits you and fits your lifestyle. If you are looking for cardiovascular benefit, you really want this to be part of your ordinary, daily routine.

It is impossible to overemphasize the importance of exercise in keeping your heart healthy. We'll discuss it at much greater length in the exercise segment of the book, so stay tuned.

Are you under stress?

Does stress increase your risk for coronary heart disease? The answer is yes. But that doesn't mean that if you are stressed out, you're necessarily going to develop it.

Different people respond to stress differently, and we think that the way you do it is the key to your stress-related heart attack risk.

You're probably familiar with the very basic personality breakdowns, type A and type B. Type As tend to fight a lot, and they attack problems aggressively. When confronted with a stressful situation, they react forcefully, and their response is very stressful for their own bodies (not just the people around them). Type-B people, on the other hand, tend to be mellower—they're more likely to experience stressful situations as temporary setbacks, or as water under the bridge. In terms of heart attack risk, type A–like people are called "hot reactors." Their blood pressure and heart rates go up dramatically when they're under pressure, while type Bs don't react as strongly.

So what can you do to reduce stress-related heart attack risk? There are two choices: Reduce the stress in your life or learn to handle the stress better. So you can try to rid your life of stress, whether that means quitting your horrible job, finding a way to make your marriage work, or moving to a smaller house so that you are living within your means. Alternatively, there are a number of well-documented techniques to handle your stress, such as breathing techniques, meditation, and my personal favorite: exercise.

Even if your stress isn't going anywhere and reduction techniques aren't getting the job done, there's still good news: You can change the way you respond to stress. In other words, even if you're a type A, you can actually turn yourself into a cold reactor, someone who reacts to stress like a type B personality. Dr. Robert Eliot did lots of excellent work on this, including the way that you can use humor to change your reaction to stress, and I wholeheartedly recommend his book *Is It Worth Dying For?* Even if you're not able to change the way you react mentally to stressful situations, you may be able to improve your physiological reactions, such as your blood pressure and heart rate levels, which will decrease your risk of heart attack.

The interesting thing about type A/type B and their relative heart attack risk: While type As are more likely to experience a first heart attack, they're *less* likely to experience a second. They tend to attack their lifestyle issues in a quintessentially aggressive type-A manner (taking up an exercise program, following a special diet, quitting smoking), whereas their type-B counterparts tend to be less proactive about making the changes that could prevent the next one.

Hopefully, by the end of this book, you'll be a cold reactor with a type-A attitude toward adopting heart-healthy lifestyle changes!

ARE YOU READY TO FIND OUT *YOUR* RISK FACTOR SCORE?

Now you're acquainted with the types of risk factors that can affect your heart health. Hopefully, you've also gained a sense of empowerment from seeing just how much control you have over these risk factors when you choose a heart-healthy lifestyle. So remember, as you take the self-assessment test to discover just what risk factors you face, *you're in control*. You can minimize the impact of the negative factors stacked against you simply by making everyday lifestyle modifications.

The self-assessment quiz you are about to take is the first step in building your Cardiac Fingerprint. Answer honestly, and rest assured: No matter what score you end up with, you have the power to change your cardiac destiny, and you will find the information you need to do so within the covers of this book.

So get your pencil ready and let's begin.

YOUR PERSONAL RISK PROFILE: SELF-ASSESSMENT QUIZ #1

ALL YOU NEED TO DO to complete your Personal Risk Profile is to answer each of the questions below and total up your points.

When you're done, your score will indicate, in a very general way, what your level of risk is for developing cardiovascular disease or heart attack.

Remember, this is not a diagnostic tool and your score is not a diagnosis! This is a tool to provide you and your doctor with a general appraisal of your risk level. It's something I use with new patients to determine if they could benefit from more sophisticated blood tests. I strongly recommend that you share your results with your personal physician at your next scheduled visit. If your test score raises any immediate questions and concerns, then call and make an appointment specifically to discuss the test and your results.

To complete your risk profile, enter the number that corresponds with the answer you choose on the line provided.

1. How old are you?

< 40　0

40–44　1

45–49　2

50–54　4

55–59　6

≥ 60　8

Your age score: _____

2. What is your gender?

Male　2

Postmenopausal female　2

Premenopausal female　0

Your gender score: _____

■ *Postmenopausal women who are taking hormone therapy should consider themselves premenopausal for the purposes of this quiz.*

3. Are you a smoker?

I currently smoke　2

I stopped smoking 1–5 years ago　1

I stopped smoking more than 5 years ago　0

I am a nonsmoker　0

I live with a smoker　1

Your smoking score: _____

4. Are you overweight?

BMI ≤ 25　0

BMI 26–29　2

BMI 30–31　4

BMI ≥ 32　6

Your body mass score: _____

■ *See the BMI chart on page 34 to determine your score.*

5. Do you have a family history of coronary heart disease?

No family history of heart disease　0

One first-degree relative with heart disease　4

Two first-degree relatives with heart disease　6

No knowledge of family history　3

Your family history score: _____

- *A first-degree relative is a mother, father, sister, or brother. Heart problems like a bad heart valve don't count.*

6. Do you know that you already have coronary heart disease?

Yes   6

No   0

Your personal heart disease score: _____

- *This includes angina, a myocardial infarction, angioplasty, stent placement, an ischemic stress test, or coronary bypass surgery.*

7. Do you have coronary ear creases on both ears?

Yes   1

No   0

Your coronary ear crease score: _____

- *A coronary ear crease is a 45-degree crease in your ears that slants upward (in the direction from your neck to your eyebrow).*

8. Do you have vertex male-pattern baldness?

Yes   1

No   0

Your vertex male-pattern baldness score: _____

- *Vertex male-pattern baldness means that you have hair on the sides but are bald on top, like Bozo the Clown.*

9. Do you have yellow-white rings circling your pupils, in the colored part of your eye (called arcus senilis)?

Yes   1

No   0

Your arcus senilis score: _____

10. Are you of Asian Indian descent?

Yes   6

No   0

Are you of Native American descent?

Yes   3

No   0

Are you of Mexican-American descent?

Yes   3

No   0

Are you of Native Hawaiian or Pacific Islander descent?

Yes   3

No   0

Your ethnicity score: _____

- *"Descent" means that at least one of your grandparents or parents is of this ethnicity.*

11. Has it been your habit to eat fish at least three times a week?

Yes   -2

No   0

Your fish consumption score: _____

12. How often do you eat red meat?

Daily   2

3–4 times a week   1

1 time a week, rarely, or never   0

Your red meat consumption score: _____

13. How often do you exercise?

6 or 7 times a week for at least 2 years   -2

4 or 5 times a week for at least 2 years   -1

3 times a week for at least 2 years   0

Less than 3 times a week for at least 2 years   1

No routine exercise   3

Your exercise score: _____

(continued)

YOUR PERSONAL RISK PROFILE: SELF-ASSESSMENT QUIZ #1 (*cont.*)

14. Are you in a high economic bracket for your geographic location?

Yes   -1

No   1

Your economic score: _____

15. Do you intentionally include fiber in your diet on a daily basis?

Yes   -1

No   0

Your fiber score: _____

16. Are you in a chronic social, work, or personal high-stress situation?

Yes   2

No   0

Your stress score: _____

17. Are you divorced (and not remarried)?

Yes   1

No   0

Your divorce score: _____

18. Have you regularly worked late-night shifts for 20 years or more?

Yes   1

No   0

Your late-night shift score: _____

19. Do you have a quick temper?

Yes   1

No   0

Your temper score: _____

20. Do you consume black or green tea on a daily basis?

Yes   -1

No   0

Your tea consumption score: _____

21. Are you taking daily aspirin therapy on your doctor's orders?

Yes   -1

No   0

Your aspirin score: _____

22. Do you have kidney disease?

Yes   2

No   0

Your kidney disease score: _____

23. Do you have diabetes mellitus?

Yes   4

No   0

Your diabetes score: _____

24. Do you have chronic oral gum disease?

Yes   1

No   0

Your gum disease score: _____

25. Do you have more than two colds or infections per year?

Yes   1

No   0

Your annual infection score: _____

26. Do you have blood type A?

    Yes   1

    No   0

    Don't know   0

Your blood type A score: _____

27. Do you have blood type O?

    Yes   -1

    No   0

    Don't know   0

Your blood type O score: _____

28. Does your mother, father, or any of your siblings have diabetes?

    Yes   2

    No   0

Your diabetes family history score: _____

29. Are you concerned that you may have an undiscovered metabolic risk for heart attack?

    Yes   2

    No   0

Your undiscovered risk concern score: _____

30. Do you have a history of high blood pressure?

    Yes—chronically and not well-controlled   4

    Yes—chronically but well-controlled   2

    Yes—but only occasionally noticed   1

    No   0

Your high blood pressure score: _____

31. Have you had your blood cholesterol tested?

    No   2

    Yes   0

Your blood cholesterol test score: _____

32. Do you have a history of high blood cholesterol?

    Yes   3

    No   0

    Don't know   0

Your blood cholesterol score: _____

33. Do you have a history of low HDL cholesterol?

    Yes   3

    No   0

    Don't know   0

Your HDL cholesterol score: _____

Your total Personal Risk Profile score: _____

YOUR CARDIAC SCORECARD

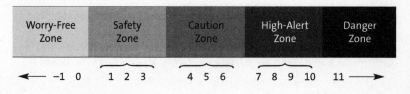

(continued)

YOUR PERSONAL RISK PROFILE: UNDERSTANDING YOUR CARDIAC SCORECARD

If your score is in the negative numbers or 0, you've landed in the Worry-Free Zone.

Almost No Risk

My hat is off to you! A final score that's a negative number might seem odd, but it's actually the best score you can get.

Your negative score lands you in the Worry-Free Zone, and that means you're probably in great cardiac shape and are likely to stay that way. Not only is it highly unlikely that you have a genetic predisposition to heart disease, but your lifestyle is also on track, which should help you stay on this heart-healthy path.

If your score is 1 to 3, you've landed in the Safety Zone.

Low Risk

Congratulations! All of the possible risk factors are breaking in your favor: Your genetic predisposition, your lifestyle, your current physical condition, and family history all are sending the risk arrow in a very heart-healthy direction! Based on this score, it's unlikely that you have any underlying metabolic imbalances that would increase your risk of having coronary heart disease. As a result, there is no immediate need for you to undergo the new cardiac screening tests for the Advanced Metabolic Markers unless your physician thinks otherwise. It never hurts, and doing so will provide you with a baseline for later comparison, but there's certainly no hurry.

You'll find lots of useful information to help you maximize your prevention efforts in part 2 of the book.

Note: You'll want to stay alert to any life changes or changes in your health that would significantly alter the answers you've given to the questions above. If any changes occur, it may be time for you to take the test again.

If your score is 4 to 6, you've landed in the Caution Zone.

Moderate Risk

Your score indicates that you very possibly have one or more of the underlying metabolic disorders that can significantly increase your risk of coronary heart disease. I'd be gambling, but I'd say there's a 50/50 chance that if you take the advanced blood tests, you'll find at least one of these Advanced Metabolic Markers for cardiovascular risk.

These disorders are dangerous when left untreated. To be on the safe side, talk to your physician about pursuing these tests now. Since there is no downside to taking the tests, I'd encourage anyone in this category to go ahead and get tested. If you were my patient, I'd strongly recommend that you do so, so we could gather the information necessary to customize a set of programs to target your specific needs. If all the test results are fine, then terrific. But if one or more are abnormal, then you have a head start on any potential heart problems.

If your score is 7 to 10, you've landed in the High-Alert Zone.
High Risk

Your score indicates a high probability that you have an underlying metabolic disorder that would increase your risk of heart attack or cardiac disease. In fact, if we were in Vegas at a craps table, I would put my money on it. With scores in this range, I'd be right more times than I'd be wrong.

My general advice to you, as it would be to any patient who came to me with this score, is to strongly suggest that you arrange to have your Advanced Metabolic Marker Profile done. It's important to find out what metabolic conditions you're dealing with so that you can counterattack immediately. The whole point of early screening is to strike the disease process before it can strike you! Once we isolate the specific risk factors you are facing, we can do something about it.

We can change your profile from high to low—or almost no—risk. Part 2 of the book is designed to help you find the individualized Nutrition, Exercise, Medication, and Supplement Prescriptions that can help you do that.

If your score is 11 to 75, you've landed in the Danger Zone.
Extreme Risk

If you scored in this range, I'd be willing to bet the mortgage on my house that you have an underlying metabolic disorder that puts you at cardiac risk; from your answers, it's almost guaranteed. You need to see your doctor as soon as possible for a complete physical and medical history. Your high score is tripping alarm bells: I strongly suggest that you consider getting the advanced blood tests done after a consultation with your personal physician.

These tests will reveal precisely what imbalances are putting you in harm's way so you and your physician can immediately begin to combat the metabolic disorders that are poised to strike your heart. This shouldn't wait. If you scored in this range, you need to make an appointment with your doctor as soon as possible to help you pursue this new generation of advanced blood tests.

You don't need to panic, you simply need to get busy. Left unattended, your situation will almost certainly lead to big trouble. But once the screening tests reveal the specific threats you are facing, we can address them through specially designed Nutrition, Exercise, Supplement, and Medication Prescriptions. With these tools at your disposal, you can literally disarm the enemy. Part 2 of this book will show you how you can take even the most extreme risk profile and turn it around.

THE NEXT STEP

You've now completed the first stage in building a Cardiac Fingerprint. Your Personal Risk Profile score determines to a large degree whether it makes sense for you now to also get the metabolic marker tests done—nothing more complicated than a simple blood test, but one than can save your life! (You'll find more information on getting these tests in chapter 5.)

As I've suggested, the decision to pursue testing is one that you and your doctor will make together, and you'll want to discuss the results of your self-test with your doctor in any event. But as a general rule, I would recommend that anyone who scores 4 or above would be well-advised to consider the advanced blood tests.

Since this is a simple blood test, there's no harm in taking it, even if there's no immediate necessity. Some people with lower scores may want to do so for the purposes of establishing a baseline, and that's fine.

For those of you who do decide to have these Advanced Metabolic Marker screening tests, the results will complete your Cardiac Fingerprint—and once your Fingerprint is complete, it will serve as your passport to the individualized programs in part 2 of the book. These test results, combined with the information we already have about you from your Personal Risk Profile, will be all the information you'll need to find the right Nutrition, Exercise, Supplement, and Medication Prescriptions to fit your cardiac profile. It's easy!

But first, in the section that follows, I'll review with you what sorts of things these tests are screening for, and why they have an impact on your cardiac health. Just as we reviewed the risk factors before taking your self-assessment test, we'll now review these Advanced Metabolic Markers. When your blood test results come back, you'll be able to complete another simple questionnaire, which will incorporate the new information from your lab results. That second questionnaire (the Advanced Metabolic Marker Profile, on page 78) will be the final step in completing your Cardiac Fingerprint.

If you will not be doing the screening tests or don't want to wait for your lab results to come back before you get started, that's just fine. Even if you don't have a complete Cardiac Fingerprint, I can direct you to a diet and exercise program that will get you started on the road to cardiac health in part 2 of the book.

4

UNLOCKING THE SECRETS OF YOUR HEART: THE NEW GENERATION OF SCREENING TESTS

THE SELF-ASSESSMENT TEST in chapter 3 has given you a general sense of where you fall in the risk gradient. If the risk arrow is pointing in a direction that suggests you might be at risk, you'll want to consider getting your blood tested for additional metabolic markers. If the risk arrow is pointing to the Danger Zone, don't waste any time! The Advanced Metabolic Marker screening tests will reveal everything you and your doctor will need to begin your counterattack, and this information will also help us to complete your Cardiac Fingerprint. Once completed, the contents of your Cardiac Fingerprint will lead you to the individualized Nutrition, Exercise, Supplement, and Medication Prescriptions in part 2 of the book, ones that are designed specifically for your unique cardiac profile.

THE LAB TESTS

Most of you are probably already familiar with the blood test that checks your cholesterol levels. Indeed, if you've seen a doctor for a physical any time in the last few years, chances are good that you've had your cholesterol levels checked. If your doctor hasn't mentioned your results, that probably means that they were normal and your doctor didn't see any need for further discussion.

When we speak of today's groundbreaking screening tests, we are referring to blood tests that offer a far more comprehensive and reliable prediction of your chances for future cardiac problems than the standard cholesterol tests alone can provide. Still, the standard cholesterol tests are one piece of that complete screening process. In other words, if you opt to have the Advanced Metabolic Marker screening tests done, your cholesterol levels will automatically be included in that battery of tests.

There is still much value to the cholesterol testing, especially since we can view it in the context of the broader puzzle. But now that we have the technology that can also measure these metabolic markers, using cholesterol numbers as our *sole* predictor of your risk of cardiac disease is sort of like doing surgery with a buzz saw. It isn't the right tool for getting the precision work done. We now have much more accurate tools: For example, one of these Advanced Metabolic Marker tests is *twice* as likely to accurately predict a heart attack as the standard cholesterol test!

Since the new screening tests include both the standard cholesterol and your Advanced Metabolic Markers, in this section I will walk you through the basics of each, explaining how each of these factors impacts your heart. The cutoff numbers in the headings that follow are the levels at which your numbers become abnormal; as you'll see, you'll need this information to find your Prescriptions in the second half of the book, but you don't have to worry about them just yet.

Since these tests and the markers they reveal will be new to most of you, and maybe even to your doctors, I feel it's important to tell you a little bit about them so that you can make sense of the results you get back. My hope is that by encouraging you to take the tests, and by clarifying what it all means, I'll help empower you to take charge of your heart health—before it is too late. I'll begin with the cholesterol tests, since those will be most familiar to you, and then move through each of the Advanced Metabolic Markers that you'll be tested for.

Otherwise known as the **standard lipid panel**, the standard cholesterol test you get when you have a physical measures total cholesterol, low-density lipoprotein cholesterol, high-density lipoprotein cholesterol, and triglycerides. Although you've almost undoubtedly had these tests done, you may not be sure what they really measure and how your test results correlate to coronary heart disease risk. Let's look at them together.

Total Cholesterol (TC)

Abnormal result: 200 milligrams per deciliter (mg/dl) or above

The standard lipid panel measures, among other things, the level of cholesterol in your blood. This is called your total cholesterol.

Despite the bad rap it's gotten, cholesterol isn't inherently bad. Your body needs it to produce cell membranes, hormones, and bile acids, as well as the material that helps keep skin moisturized. Cholesterol comes from two sources: Our liver produces 60 to 80 percent of what we need and we get some from the foods that we eat.

Cholesterol is carried in several different types of lipoprotein balls that package the fatty cholesterol so that it can travel through the bloodstream, which is essentially water. Otherwise, the cholesterol would just float to the top, like the fat in chicken soup.

In the 1950s, John William Gofman, Ph.D., M.D., and his colleagues at the University of California at Berkeley discovered that when they put blood into a centrifuge, the lipoproteins in it float at different levels according to their density. Gofman's research is among the most significant developments of the last 50 years. We now know that these different-density lipoproteins behave very differently in the bloodstream and that their size is directly correlated to your risk of coronary artery disease.

Chylomicrons, also lipoproteins, are huge balls carrying triglycerides and relatively little cholesterol. These are produced in the intestines and increase dramatically after a fatty meal. **Very low-density lipoprotein (VLDL)** is also large and rich in triglycerides, but it is produced in the liver. **Low-density lipoprotein** (LDL), which is often known as "bad" cholesterol, is rich in cholesterol with few triglycerides. **Intermediate-density lipoprotein** (IDL) is the size between VLDL and LDL. **High-density lipoprotein** (HDL), known as "good" cholesterol, is also primarily a cholesterol carrier (although it's carrying that cholesterol in the direction opposite of the way the LDL carries its load).

I *prefer* to see total cholesterol well below this cutoff, around 140 mg/dl.

LDL Cholesterol (LDL-C)

Abnormal result: 130 milligrams per deciliter (mg/dl) or above

LDL cholesterol, the "bad" cholesterol, carries cholesterol from the liver to cells in the body. High levels of it contribute to the risk of coronary artery disease, and it is one of the primary markers used to predict coronary artery disease.

As LDL passes through the arteries, it can get trapped in already existing lesions. There, it's prone to oxidization, which further damages the arteries. Like many of the markers for coronary heart disease, a predisposition toward high LDL can be inherited. This condition is called **familial hypercholesterolemia** (FH) and is often found in people with very elevated total cholesterol. People with this condition have inherited one or more defective genes, which means they can't clear LDL cholesterol from the bloodstream as well as people with both genes intact can. This leads to elevated LDL cholesterol in the blood. FH is associated with dramatically high levels of premature atherosclerosis (three or four times higher than normal), so if you have high LDL cholesterol, lifestyle changes and medication will substantially decrease your risk of developing coronary heart disease.

You can lower LDL cholesterol in four ways: by decreasing the amount of saturated fat you consume in food; by inhibiting the absorption of cholesterol in foods; by inhibiting the body's ability to produce cholesterol; and by increasing the body's ability to metabolize it, so that it's taken out of the bloodstream in higher quantities.

The first one is self-explanatory. Decrease the amount of dietary cholesterol you take in and you'll see a decrease in your blood cholesterol. In the Nutrition Prescription in part 2 of the book, we'll give you a list of foods that contain cholesterol so you can avoid them.

If your LDL problem is severe, medication is the right path to take. Other types of medication, including the bile acid–binding resins, can help prevent the absorption of cholesterol. The statin drugs inhibit the body's production of cholesterol: They block the body's ability to make cholesterol. We'll talk about this in greater detail in the medication chapter.

Increasing the body's ability to metabolize cholesterol is a little more complicated. There are docking sites in the liver called LDL receptors. When blood cholesterol is low and the liver needs extra cholesterol to perform essential functions, it increases these LDL receptors so that they remove more LDL cholesterol from the blood. There are medications that do this, as well.

Foods high in saturated fats (meat, full-fat dairy products, lard, and coconut and palm oils) are bad not only because they contain a lot of cholesterol and saturated fats, but also because they encourage the suppression of these LDL receptors, which means that the liver is removing cholesterol less efficiently from the bloodstream. Some of the metabolic disorders that we'll discuss in this chapter exacerbate this, and it can really become a problem.

Anything over 130 mg/dl is abnormal and should be considered an alert. The National Institutes of Health's Cholesterol Education Program, which periodically releases its recommendations for cholesterol levels, suggests that you should keep LDL cholesterol below 100, and I agree that that should be your goal.

A word of warning: LDL tends to be the number people focus on when they get their test results. It's an important number, especially if you have a classic lipid disorder, but it's also very important to remember that a good LDL number does not in any way guarantee heart health. A great number of people with LDL below 100 end up in cardiac care units.

HDL Cholesterol (HDL-C)

Abnormal result: 40 milligrams per deciliter (mg/dl) or below in men and postmenopausal women; 50 milligrams per deciliter (mg/dl) or below in premenopausal women and women on hormone therapy

HDL is called the "good" cholesterol because high levels of it are correlated to a reduced risk of coronary artery disease. HDL removes cholesterol away from the artery walls (including from plaque) and carries it back to the liver for reprocessing, where it is either recycled or excreted. This process is called **reverse cholesterol transport** (RCT). HDL also carries an important natural antioxidant enzyme, one that prevents the damaging oxidization of LDL cholesterol.

I love to see HDL above 60 in premenopausal women, above 50 in men and postmenopausal women, and even higher if I discover that you have another one of these metabolic markers. You can raise HDL cholesterol a number of ways (all of which we'll discuss later in the book): Loss of excess body fat is key; vigorous exercise is another way to drive those values up. Various medications can also help.

Triglycerides (TG)

Abnormal result: 140 milligrams per deciliter (mg/dl) or above

The other test done as part of the standard lipid panel is a measure of triglycerides. When you eat, your body converts extra energy into a form of energy that can be stored for later use. So calories get turned into fats, and when three of these fats are stuck together, they're called triglycerides (*tri-* means three).

Too many triglycerides in the bloodstream is called **hypertriglyceridemia**. Triglycerides have been linked to both coronary and peripheral artery disease, independent of LDL levels, and high levels are strong predictors of heart attack. High triglycerides are especially worrisome when they're found in combination with high LDL cholesterol.

I like to see triglycerides in my patients around 70, and since diet is extremely important in controlling triglycerides, that's within most people's reach if they're paying attention to what they eat. Since triglycerides can be the result of extra sugar in the blood, eating too many carbohydrates and simple sugars (and alcohol) can result in elevated levels. Diets high in saturated fats can also contribute. Losing excess body weight can be powerful in controlling them.

Why isn't the standard cholesterol test enough?

Since the 1980s, physicians have based their assessment of your coronary heart disease risk on the results of the standard cholesterol test.

It is certainly true that the higher the cholesterol, the greater the likelihood of coronary heart disease. So when the number is very high, this can be a very useful test. But it's not a particularly refined test, and it certainly isn't foolproof. It's only an indicator for one genetic abnormality. If these were reliable predictors, I wouldn't be seeing so many people in my clinic with "normal" standard lipid panels—and positive coronary calcification tests indicating that they already have significant arterial damage. Or people with a history of "normal" lipid panels, wondering what could have caused their first heart attack.

Focusing exclusively on the high blood cholesterol issue means that we're ignoring 50 to 80 percent of the people who will develop coronary heart disease. For many people, this test will simply not catch their cardiac problem. A set of normal cholesterol results doesn't mean that you can rest easy. Cholesterol is just one part of a much bigger picture, one that includes a host of metabolic factors that directly increase your risk of developing coronary heart disease and experiencing a cardiac event. In order to outwit your genes, we need to isolate and measure other indicators. Let's take a look at those other factors.

THE ADVANCED METABOLIC MARKERS

Although the names of these metabolic markers won't be as familiar to you as cholesterol is, some of these new markers have been making headlines in magazines such as Scientific American's *Medicine*, *Men's Health*, *Time*, *Reader's Digest*, *Esquire*, and others. Fortunately, as more and more studies are being reported in the medical journals with results too important to ignore, the news is getting out there. And it's about time!

THE NEW GENERATION OF SCREENING TESTS

SMALL LDL

A small, dense, and very dangerous form of LDL cholesterol. People with a large number of these small LDLs are called **LDL pattern B** and carry a much higher risk of coronary heart disease and heart attack.

APOLIPOPROTEIN B (APO B)

A much more accurate way of measuring the *number* of LDLs in your blood—not just the amount of cholesterol. This alerts us to the presence of those small, dangerous LDLs.

HDL2B

The subclass of HDL that offers the greatest level of protection for your heart. You can't have too much of it!

HIGH-SENSITIVITY C-REACTIVE PROTEIN (HS-CRP)

A telling sign of inflammation—and *twice* as likely to predict heart attack as LDL.

FIBRINOGEN

Promotes blood clots, a contributing factor in many heart attacks.

CHLAMYDIA PNEUMONIAE

A relatively harmless bacterium with serious consequences for your heart.

INSULIN

Elevated levels of this hormone have been linked to coronary heart disease—and when it's detected in combination with some of these other markers, it can mean real trouble.

HOMOCYSTEINE

A natural and harmless amino acid by-product, produced and eliminated by the body—unless you've inherited an inability to metabolize it. In this case, levels can become too high, putting you at serious risk.

LIPOPROTEIN (A) [LP(A)]

High levels increase your risk 300 percent, even if everything else is normal.

APOLIPOPROTEIN E (APO E)

A real indicator of risk—and a test that tells how well you'll respond to dietary changes.

The truly terrific news: When your metabolic marker tests reveal an imbalance, it can almost always be treated. This is why I believe that most heart attacks are preventable: We can now home in on your specific metabolic issues, devise a customized action plan, and treat your (present or future) cardiac problem at its source. So after you've been tested, you'll be able to find the individualized Prescription plans in part 2 to enable you to outsmart your genes.

Who should get the Advanced Metabolic Marker tests?
- Anyone who scored 4 or above on their Personal Risk Profile
- Anyone with coronary heart disease

If you scored 4 or above on the Personal Risk Profile, then you're at fairly high risk for developing coronary heart disease as a result of an undiscovered metabolic condition. This isn't to say that you *have* one of these metabolic conditions, just that your genes and your lifestyle are conspiring to increase your risk. The additional information that you and your physician can gather from these tests may give you the ability to swerve to avoid future trouble instead of crashing into it head on, and I recommend that you pursue these tests.

But what if your cholesterol numbers are normal?
It doesn't matter. If your Personal Risk Profile score is high, you should still get the tests. We've reviewed how a normal set of results from the standard cholesterol tests doesn't mean that you can rest easy. Remember all those "stealth" heart attacks? Those people thought they were in the clear, too. Cholesterol is only part of the puzzle. You might still have an undiagnosed disorder that's putting you at risk.

You're already taking medication to control your cholesterol. Do you still need the tests?
Yes. Even if you're already addressing your cholesterol problem, it doesn't mean that there aren't other underlying conditions also affecting your heart health. If your assessment score was high, it's time for you to find out

what's really going on. If it turns out that you do have metabolic imbalances along with the high cholesterol you already know about, that puts you at even higher risk. So it's *especially* important for people with abnormal cholesterol to find out if there are any additional factors contributing to their risk.

Here are the metabolic markers that are included in the advanced screening tests.

Small LDL: Pattern A or Pattern B?

Abnormal result: 257 angstroms or below

LDL IIIa + IIIb at 20 percent or above

One of the most important refinements we've been able to make on the standard cholesterol test is in the area of LDL. The standard cholesterol test measures the general amount of LDL cholesterol in your system, and that's useful. But when we drill down to the next level, we discover that there are a number of different kinds of LDL cholesterol, with radically diverse effects on your risk profile.

In the case of LDL, size really does matter. The presence of a large number of a particular kind of LDL, an especially small, dense kind, where particles measure less than 257 angstroms, is one of the most serious indicators for coronary heart disease that we can measure. If you have a lot of this small, dense LDL, we say that you're an **LDL pattern B**. (People whose LDL is predominantly large are called **LDL pattern A**.) This piece of information is one of the most powerful determinants in your Cardiac Fingerprint; as you'll see, if you are LDL pattern B, you are at a dramatically increased risk for coronary heart disease.

Pattern B and Increased Risk

Small LDL (or ALP, for atherogenic lipoprotein profile) is what we call an **independent marker** for coronary heart disease. This means that you're still at serious risk from this dangerous LDL, even if everything else (like your body weight and your standard cholesterol test) is perfect.

And the risk from this small LDL is quite significant. People who have small LDL are *three times* more likely to have coronary artery disease; worse, that risk doubles to *six* times if you have a lot of these LDL particles.

These two factors—the fact that this small LDL increases your risk even if you look great in all other respects, and the degree to which it increases your risk—go a long way toward explaining a lot of those "stealth" heart attacks, doesn't it? And since we can now test for it and treat it, it means that the majority of those stealth heart attacks are preventable.

A *lot* of people have inherited this LDL pattern B trait, which is another

> People with small LDL, also known as LDL pattern B, are three times more likely to have coronary artery disease. People with a lot of it see their risk increase to six times the normal level.

reason it heads our list of red alerts. According to a Boston area health study, 50 percent of men and 30 percent of premenopausal women with coronary heart disease express this small LDL disorder. Small LDL does tend to show up more in people who have a high-carbohydrate diet, have gained a lot of weight, and who don't exercise. It often occurs in people who are overweight or diabetic, for example, and in those whose tests show high triglycerides. But it's a hereditary disorder, and it also occurs *often* in the perfectly fit, so it's a useful risk indicator for everyone, regardless of your physical condition.

Small Particle, Big Damage

Why is this tiny lipoprotein such a big deal?

First of all, the size of these particles makes it easier for them to weasel their way up into the artery wall, where they cause all kinds of damage. And the presence of small LDL also implies the presence of a truly nasty metabolic stew. The stew includes rapid progression of partially blocked arteries; arteries that are more prone to sudden spasm; an increased number of blood fats after a meal; lousy removal of cholesterol from the blood supply; increased likelihood of oxidation and susceptibility to oxidative damage; blood factors that increase the likelihood of a heart attack caused by a blood clot; insulin resistance; and plaque instability—to name a few. In other words, small LDL predicts most of the truly terrible things that can happen to your heart.

You may not have all of these things if you have small LDL, but they're all associated with it, and you're more likely to suffer from them if you have small LDL. People with small LDL are also more likely to have low HDL, or "good" cholesterol, which means that cholesterol isn't taken out of artery blockages as well and as fast as it might be. Low HDL is also associated with an increased risk of cardiovascular disease.

So those are some of the very good reasons that we worry so much about catching and treating small LDL.

The Small LDL Paradox

There's another reason we want to be aggressive about catching and treating small LDL, and that's the paradox associated with it. If you have small LDL and have coronary heart disease, your disease will get worse twice as fast as it will in someone who doesn't have small LDL. But if you treat it, you can seriously retard the further development of the blockages and in many cases stop the progression of the disease more easily than can someone who doesn't have these small particles. In fact, in a small percentage of cases, you can actually cause the disease to regress. In other words, **LDL pattern B patients have the most rapidly progressive disease, but they are also the patients who respond best to treatment.** So if we get you early, we have a really good shot at making you better. For this reason, it's really in our best interest to catch and treat this condition without wasting time.

Catching Small LDL Early

Your family provides you with yet another reason to find out if you're LDL pattern B. Remember, this small LDL trait is inherited. This means that if one of your parents have it, you and your siblings each had a 50 percent chance of inheriting it. So if you test positive for an abundance of this small LDL, you might suggest to your primary relatives (parents, siblings, children) that they get tested as well. The results of your blood test could prevent your father's second heart attack! And since this problem is so directly affected by lifestyle choices such as diet and exercise, we love to catch this one early, way before serious damage occurs. For instance, if we determine that your son is also pattern B while he's still in his twenties, he'll have a real head start on making appropriate lifestyle adjustments before he runs into serious heart trouble later.

Small LDL Multiplies Other Risk Factors

If you're not yet convinced, here's another reason to find out if you're pattern B: As we saw in that metabolic stew, small LDL may act as an indicator for other problems. It's often a precursor for type 2 diabetes. People with small LDL may also have even greater heart disease risk if they also have high homocysteine, apo B, and Lp(a) (we'll discuss these in more depth in a minute), which have all been linked to increased rates of coronary artery disease.

So if you discover that you're prone to this trait, it alerts you and your doctor to stay vigilant for some of the other health problems that traditionally accompany it. In fact, a combination of risk markers can *multiply* your risk of coronary artery disease. Other markers are especially dangerous when they're found with small LDL. People with small LDL may also have elevated apo B, for example, and a study in Quebec determined that the risk of coronary artery disease increased by *six times* when high levels of small LDL were combined with elevated apo B. Elevated blood insulin levels are also a coronary heart disease risk factor by themselves. However, the presence of all three: small LDL, elevated apo B, and elevated resting insulin ratchets your risk up to an alarming 20 times normal.

This is a good illustration of the way that these more sophisticated tests can catch individuals who are at tremendously elevated risk, when they might otherwise have slipped through the cracks. So your doctor can use this information very constructively in determining how aggressively you should pursue treatment. If you have a number of these disorders, your risk skyrockets and you'll know to take a hard line on treatment.

Small LDL Is Treatable

Here's some good news: Although the size of your LDL particles is genetically determined, your risk can definitely be modified through treatment.

In fact, we can actually convert you from a high-risk LDL pattern B to a low-risk LDL pattern A! And the treatment isn't complicated or expensive. In fact, weight control, a diet relatively low in saturated fat and simple sugars, and an adequate amount of exercise will do the trick (with some drugs such as fibrates and nicotinic acid, or niacin, thrown in if the problem is severe). People who are LDL pattern B tend to respond very well to treatment, so if you have this risk factor, don't despair. Just get busy!

There's one more reason it's good to know if you're pattern B: If you're not, your super-low-fat diet may make you one! It's true: While diets low in saturated fat are often very effective in converting LDL pattern B to LDL pattern A, if a diet is *too low* in fat, it can cause the more harmless pattern As to convert into the much more pernicious pattern B, if those As have the genetic potential but aren't yet expressing it. As you'll see in the Nutrition Prescription, we don't recommend that people who are pattern A drop their fat below 25 percent of their total calories.

What the Twin Peaks Mean

When you get your lab results back, you'll see that LDL pattern B is represented by a graph with at least one spiky peak, indicating whether the majority of the LDL are small or large. The ranges are as follows: from 263.5 to 285, particles are considered to be large. From 257.5 to 263.4, the particles are intermediate. And from 220 to 257.4, they're considered small. The peaks indicate which size bracket the majority of your particles fall into.

About 40 percent of people have more than one peak when their results come back, which indicates that they have both small and large LDL particles. If the taller peak is in the larger range, you're LDL pattern A. If the taller peak is in the smaller range, you're LDL pattern B. Because you can change the size of the particles, these dual peaks give you a good indication of your conversion potential. If your bigger peak is in the larger area, but there's a smaller peak lurking in the pattern B area, you know that you have to be vigilant about the lifestyle issues that can push you toward the production of more small and dangerous LDL. If your big peak is in the small LDL area, but you have a smaller peak in the large LDL area, that gives you something to work toward. If you're good about diet and exercise (and medication, if that's the path you and your doctor have decided is right for you), you should be able to watch the peaks even out as your LDL redistributes itself, until finally the peak in the small area is completely gone.

The peaks give you and your doctor a good indication that you're responding well to your therapy. It's gratifying, and it's not very hard. I've seen people move from LDL pattern B to pattern A with nothing more than a 10-pound weight loss!

Ideally, we'd like to see you with very few or no LDL particles measuring less than 263 angstroms.

Beyond pattern B?

In fact, these peaks allow us to go *beyond* the LDL pattern A and B distinctions by allowing us to look at the distribution of your LDL subclasses. The very tiny LDL subclasses, IIIa and IIIb, are independently associated with disease in the carotid arteries, and the even-smaller LDL IVb may be associated with plaque instability. If we see that a large percentage of your LDL is not only small, but concentrated in these danger zones, we know that you're at much higher risk for disease. The distribution of the small LDL you have then gives us a much more accurate picture of the risk you face from these particles.

In fact, it may alter the way we categorize you. Let's say that 50 percent of your LDL are large, so your tallest peak is in the large region, making you a pattern A. But when we look at the remainder of your LDL, we find that 30 percent is in the very dangerous LDL IIIa + IIIb region. This added risk means that we're best to treat you as a pattern B, even though you're technically a lower-risk pattern A. Anything more than 20 percent in the IIIa + IIIb regions is cause for concern, although we'd like to see that number even lower.

Apo B: A More Accurate LDL Measurement
Abnormal result: 80 milligrams per deciliter (mg/dl) or above

Our new awareness of the importance of small LDL is one of the reasons we test for **apolipoprotein B**, or apo B.

Apo B is a surface protein "cap" on the LDL particle, a protein that rides along the outside of the VLDL, IDL, and LDL particles. The LDL looks like a sphere with cholesterol stuffed inside and the apo B woven into the surface. There's only one apo B on each LDL that the liver secretes. Since there's exactly one apo B to one LDL particle, apo B is a more direct and accurate way of measuring the total LDL number than LDL-C, the standard test.

Why? Because standard LDL-C measurement is done indirectly. As the C implies, it measures the portion of the total blood cholesterol that is carried in the LDL molecule, rather than the actual number of LDLs present in the blood. We have to know *how many* LDLs someone has in their blood, not just how much cholesterol there is, to determine whether or not that person is pattern B. As you'll remember, a lot of these small LDL particles will turn a threefold risk into a sixfold risk.

Let's say that Jackie and Sue have the same amount of LDL cholesterol, so their LDL-C numbers are the same. But that number is deceptive because it conceals a greater truth: Jackie is carrying her cholesterol load on 50 large LDLs, which makes her an LDL pattern A. We know this because she has 50 apo Bs. Sue, on the other hand, has 100 apo Bs, which means she's carrying that same cholesterol load on 100 small LDLs. That puts her into the much more dangerous LDL pattern B category. These two people look identical if you're just looking at their LDL-C numbers; it's only when we count the apo Bs that we realize Sue is at a 300 percent greater risk.

In fact, the combination of "normal" LDL-C and elevated apo B may indicate that you have (wait for the mouthful) **hyperapobetalipoproteinemia**. In the Quebec study, this combination of small LDL and elevated apo B increased coronary artery disease risk sixfold.

A Threat on Its Own

There are other reasons to test for apo B. First and foremost, it is itself a coronary heart disease risk factor.

Apo B is particularly dangerous because it's this protein that gets changed when LDL becomes oxidized. The form that oxidized apo B turns into makes it much more attractive—like chocolate candy—to the scavenger receptors on the white blood cells. The white blood cells eat tons of these oxidized LDLs, then they explode, and their contents contribute to the unstable plaque that's the culprit behind so many cardiac events.

So a lot of apo B in your bloodstream means that you're at higher risk particularly if you are LDL pattern B. I like to see apo B between 40 and 60 mg/dl in my patients.

HDL2b: Taking HDL to the Next Level

Abnormal result: 35 percent of total HDL or below (premenopausal women and women on hormone therapy)

20 percent of total HDL or below (men and postmenopausal women)

Doctors have been testing for HDL for years, and a high level of HDL generally means a degree of protection from coronary heart disease. But now, just as with LDL, we also know that there are different *kinds* of HDL and they're not all created equal. Some types, or subclasses, of HDL really do protect you from coronary heart disease, and some are less useful. So your cholesterol test can come back with a very "good" HDL-C level, but without going to the next level in testing, you can't tell whether that means you're protected.

The subclass we look at most closely is called HDL2b because it's the one most strongly associated with decreased coronary artery disease risk. Here's another clue in the mystery of the stealth heart attack: You can have a high HDL-C number and still be deficient in this highly protective subclass. So your HDL numbers can look terrific on a lab report, but they're not protecting your heart. And that leaves you walking around thinking everything's fine instead of taking simple measures to increase this powerful cardiac safeguard.

What's special about HDL2b?

HDL2b is the crucial measure of **reverse cholesterol transport**, the process by which cholesterol is removed from the arteries. When you have low levels of HDL2b, cholesterol doesn't get reabsorbed as efficiently—and we know that's not good. HDL2b has another defensive weapon in its arsenal: It harbors an important natural antioxidant called **paraoxanase**, which protects the arterial cell walls.

Because it contributes so strongly to reverse cholesterol transport and because it carries this antioxidant, HDL2b has a powerfully protective effect on the heart, which increases when high levels of it are present.

When it comes to this marker, you can't have too much!

Who has low HDL2b?

There's no hard and fast rule about the kind of person likely to have low HDL2b. It's often the situation for pattern B people, but not always: It can also be low in people whose LDLs are large. An HDL2b deficit is often common in Asian-Indian patients and type 2 diabetics, so people in those groups should be extra vigilant. Smoking lowers HDL2b levels drastically. Low levels are also often found in sedentary or very overweight individuals.

Raising HDL2b

You can raise low HDL2b with a little effort, and I strongly encourage my patients to do so. I'll show *you* how to go about it in part 2.

This HDL subclass can generally be improved through changes to the diet and lifestyle: Cutting simple sugars and alcohol can help, as can weight loss, a healthy diet, and regular exercise. People who are more resistant can improve it with medications such as niacin and fibrates. Postmenopausal women with coronary heart disease who have had difficulty with medications may also want to consult with their gynecologists about hormone therapy (HT).

Because of HLD2b's incredibly powerful protective capabilities, I try to get it as high as I can in my patients, especially when they're coping with a number of these other abnormal metabolic issues. I want to see HDL2b at more than 45 percent in my premenopausal female patients and those on HT and above 35 percent in men and postmenopausal women. Again, this marker puts a mighty arrow in our quiver, but we can't use it as protection against coronary heart disease if we don't test for it.

High-Sensitivity C-Reactive Protein: A Better Indicator Than Cholesterol?

Abnormal result: 0.4 milligrams per deciliter (mg/dl) or above

Another very powerful arrow in our cardiological quiver is the test for **C-reactive protein** (CRP). (In order to detect small but medically important amounts of CRP, a high-sensitivity laboratory measure is used, so you may see this referred to as high-sensitivity CRP, or hs-CRP.)

Hs-CRP is a protein released into the bloodstream whenever there is serious inflammation in the body. We use the term **acute phase reactant** to describe any protein the body releases rapidly after it receives some kind of inflammatory insult. These acute phase reactants are designed to help the body fight back. As we know, atherosclerosis is itself a chronic, low-grade state of inflammation, so the presence of inflammation can alert us to serious and ongoing arterial damage. High levels of hs-CRP send up a flare, drawing our attention to that damage.

In fact, elevated hs-CRP is one of the best indicators we have of increased risk for coronary heart disease. People with high hs-CRP are at four to seven times more risk than people with normal levels, which may be due in part to inflammation.

Hs-CRP is a statistically significant predictor of heart attack, stroke, and recurrent coronary events. In fact, it's better, according to some studies, than the standard cholesterol tests we've been using. In a study done with 28,000

A SECRET WEAPON

- People with high hs-CRP are at four to seven times more risk than people with normal levels.

- Hs-CRP is twice as likely to predict a heart attack as high levels of LDL cholesterol are.

- Between 20 and 30 million Americans may have high hs-CRP, although their cholesterol numbers are within normal range.

women, elevated hs-CRP was *twice* as likely to predict a heart attack as high levels of LDL cholesterol were. Here's a chilling statistic: 20 to 30 million Americans may have elevated hs-CRP—and cholesterol numbers well within the acceptable range. And yet this test, with its astonishing capacity to predict cardiac event, is not yet part of the roster of routine diagnostic procedures.

Predicting a first heart attack isn't even the extent of this extraordinary test's capabilities: Hs-CRP also predicts people who won't do well after surgery, and people at high risk for another heart attack. While germs have been linked to heart attack risk, it's the combination of tests telling us you've had a recent infection and elevated hs-CRP that really helps identify people at high risk for additional coronary artery disease.

A Lighter Shade of Pale

So hs-CRP is an impressive indicator of risk. Unfortunately, it's a difficult tool to figure out how to use clinically. One of the reasons it's so tricky is that there's a huge variation in hs-CRP levels among people. In fact, there can be huge variation in hs-CRP levels in one single person over the course of a few days. Hs-CRP simply measures inflammation in the body, not specifically inflammation in your coronary arteries. Your high hs-CRP level might mean that you have coronary heart disease, but it might also mean that you're recovering from a cold or that you stepped off the curb the wrong way and stressed your knee on your way to the doctor's office.

Because hs-CRP is difficult to use in isolation, we like to look at it in combination with other risk factors. The same way a very good cook will automatically adjust a recipe to compensate for various changes in altitude or ingredients, a very good physician can use hs-CRP to inform the way he looks at the rest of your Cardiac Fingerprint.

So if you're pattern B and your hs-CRP isn't alarming, we might feel more comfortable waiting to see how you respond to a program of diet and exercise. But if you're pattern B and your hs-CRP also comes back high a number of times, we'll go after you with more proactive therapies, such as medication. Ideally, you'd test completely negative, but I'm usually satisfied to see it below 0.2 mg/dl in my patients.

As we move from the one-size-fits-all model of medicine to one where more variable factors are taken into account, hs-CRP is an incredibly valuable instrument. It gives us more of the information we need to treat each patient individually.

Is hs-CRP treatable?

We're working on treatments to lower hs-CRP. Some of those treatments may include statin drugs, fibrates (another lipid drug), and good old niacin. Aspirin doesn't lower hs-CRP, but it does have an anti-inflammatory effect of its own.

Beyond hs-CRP

An interesting note: There was an ambitious study of coronary heart disease called the West of Scotland Coronary Prevention Study and in that study, the researchers looked at another inflammatory marker called **phospholipase A2** (PLA2) in the blood samples they took. It's a much better, less volatile indicator than hs-CRP, but we don't use it yet. Why? Because there's a commercial machine available that measures hs-CRP and nothing yet to measure PLA2 except in research laboratories. Until there is, we'll continue to look at hs-CRP.

Fibrinogen: The Clotting Factor

Abnormal result: 400 milligrams per deciliter (mg/dl) or above

Another acute phase reactant, **fibrinogen** is a protein that comes to the rescue when the body gets hurt. Fibrinogen plays a role in the normal process of blood clotting. When you have a cut, this protein layers itself in filaments like string, eventually causing a kind of net or lattice that plugs up the hole. We know that thrombosis, or blood clot, at the site of ruptured plaque is one of the causes of heart attack. Elevated fibrinogen indicates that your blood is more prone to clotting.

High fibrinogen is an independent risk factor and an acute phase reactant, but we're not sure how directly coronary heart disease is correlated to it. In studies using certain cardiac drugs where cardiac disease has been reduced, fibrinogen has also been reduced. But the results aren't necessarily conclusive because other changes have occurred in those patients as well. Is the reduced coronary heart disease a result of better fibrinogen levels, or something else—like better HDL2b, for instance?

Like hs-CRP, fibrinogen is most useful when we look at it in the context of the rest of your Cardiac Fingerprint and let it help us determine how aggressively we'll treat the other metabolic issues we find. For instance, if your fibrinogen is high and you're LDL pattern B, we'll be more aggressive in treating the small LDL issue.

Treating High Fibrinogen

High fibrinogen, or **hyperfibrinogenemia**, can be inherited, but as you'll see in part 2, like so many of these inherited markers, it can be treated. Lifestyle issues are key: Smoking and obesity increase fibrinogen levels, and controlling those factors by quitting smoking and losing weight can substantially lower levels. There are reports that one of the statin drugs may raise fibrinogen as well, although this is uncommon. We do know that fibrate drugs and niacin lower fibrinogen, so your doctor may choose to use these medications (or use them in combination with a statin drug) to treat your other metabolic issues, such as low HDL. Hormone therapy in postmenopausal women decreases fibrinogen levels, but the risks of that treatment might outweigh the benefits.

Chlamydia Pneumoniae: Is That Cough Causing Your Coronary Heart Disease?

Abnormal result: 1 part in 32 parts or above

Another one of the markers we test for is an infection called *Chlamydia pneumoniae*, a fairly common bacterium that causes respiratory infections such as pneumonia.

What can the bacterium that causes bronchitis possibly have to do with heart attack? In fact, we're not really sure. No conclusive study has yet been done to prove that there's a direct relationship. There was, however, a study done in London on patients who had **atherectomy** (a procedure where a surgeon uses a cutting catheter to whittle away plaque buildup in the arteries and then sucks the resulting debris out). This study showed evidence that this germ had been present in the plaque at some point in the relatively recent past. And another study done in London with coronary heart disease patients whose blood tests showed a high level of the Chlamydia bacterium showed on two separate occasions that there was a significant reduction in future heart attacks among patients who were treated for the infection with antibiotics. Other studies in less seriously infected people have not been as successful, so it may partly be a question of how serious—or how chronic—the infection you have is.

Chlamydia is very frequently found in hospitals, which is why we see it so often in hospital workers and their regular patients. It's also common among smokers and others prone to chronic bronchial infections. You may remember that in the Personal Risk Profile, we were interested in knowing if you'd experienced two or more infections (of the urinary tract, respiratory system, etc.) a year. Recent studies have indicated that people who have a high pathogen load (who have had a lot of chronic infections) are at higher risk for coronary heart disease.

Here's what we think is happening: If you have an infection in the artery wall, then the body is chronically trying to kill that infection and repair the damage. The white blood cells are moving in, getting obese and exploding, and they're contributing to the damage. And the small LDL passing through the artery at its regular rate is suddenly finding it much easier to get up into those damaged artery walls. So instead of being absorbed at a reasonable 10 particles a minute, let's say, the number of small LDLs getting absorbed into the artery wall skyrockets to 100 particles a minute. That's how a relatively harmless chronic infection can seriously contribute to your chances of coronary heart disease.

Since the treatment for chlamydia is a simple course of antibiotics—a relatively short-term, inexpensive treatment with few side effects—we treat this infection when we see it, unless there's another contraindication.

Insulin: What's Blood Sugar Got to Do with It?
Abnormal result: 12 milliunits per milliliter (mU/ml) or above

As you may know, insulin is a regulatory hormone released by the pancreas. It ensures that your blood sugar levels stay even instead of spiking and falling dramatically depending on your food intake.

You're probably familiar with insulin in connection with the disease diabetes. Deficient insulin release is the classic cause of diabetes; diabetics have to monitor and control their own blood sugar and insulin levels because their bodies aren't doing it for them.

Insulin Resistance

There's another prediabetic condition called insulin resistance, and in most cases, this is what we're testing for. The test for elevated insulin, which is called a **glucose tolerance test**, is like a treadmill test for your pancreas. We test your fasting insulin, give you a sugar drink, and test you 2 hours later. If your insulin level is still sky-high, that indicates insulin resistance.

Here's how insulin resistance works: You eat something and your pancreas releases insulin. If your cells are resistant to the insulin, your blood sugar stays relatively high. In response, your pancreas makes more insulin, and more, and more because it takes a lot more to get the job done. Eventually, your body isn't able to keep up with the demand for insulin, and the condition turns into diabetes.

Insulin and Coronary Heart Disease

You want to know if you're insulin resistant because it tells you not only whether you're at risk for developing diabetes, but also whether you're at risk for developing coronary heart disease.

Elevated insulin levels have been linked to an increased risk of coronary artery disease, and almost all diabetics die of heart disease. Of course, insulin resistance and diabetes are often associated with overweight, which is always bad for your heart. And the hormone insulin itself is atherogenic. It stimulates smooth muscle growth and irritates the insides of the arteries. In the past 2 years, there has been a series of papers linking elevated insulin levels to **restenosis** (or further blockage) after angioplasty surgery or coronary artery stent placement surgery.

> **High insulin + high apo B + LDL pattern B increases your risk of coronary artery disease by 20 times.**

High insulin is also often linked to other lipoprotein abnormalities such as small LDL, and as we know, it can be devastating combined with some of these other markers: High insulin combined with elevated apo B and small LDL increases your risk of coronary artery disease by 20 times.

Helping Your Body to Regulate Itself

I encourage my patients to get their insulin to less than 8 mU/ml. There are two basic ways to control insulin resistance. In a healthy person without coronary heart disease, I'd recommend avoiding sugars, losing body fat if necessary, and exercising every day. Insulin works better when people lose excess body weight, so 90 percent of healthy people can control their insulin resistance through weight control. If you're lean and mean, you can usually supply enough insulin to control glucose.

Some insulin-resistant people don't respond well to lifestyle changes and are typically prone to type 2 diabetes. They've already gotten themselves into great shape and don't overdo sugar in their diets, but their bodies still can't control glucose levels, and that indicates that there's an underlying problem. With these people, we need to think about medications sooner rather than later, especially if there's already evidence of coronary heart disease.

Homocysteine, or How Spinach Can Save Your Life
Abnormal result: 14 micromoles per liter (μmol/L) or above

In 1962, a physician in Ireland studying a group of severely retarded children noticed that they all had very high levels of a naturally occurring amino acid called **homocysteine**. These children had something else in common: They had astronomically high rates of premature coronary heart disease and often died of heart attacks at ages as young as 10 years old.

Homocysteine is a naturally occurring substance, the by-product of the amino acid methionine. It's usually made after a meal rich in animal proteins and cleaned out of the bloodstream as a matter of course. Unfortunately, some people inherit an impaired ability to tidy up after themselves. Usually this inability only comes from one parent, and the body is able to compensate. But if the gene comes from both sides, homocysteine levels may grow extremely high, causing heart attacks in young children.

Clearly, these Irish children had inherited an inability to clean up their own homocysteine, and there was a link between the high levels of this amino acid in their bloodstreams and their premature heart disease. Fortunately, it's rare to get a bad gene from both parents, but getting one good one and one bad one is not uncommon.

> High homocysteine levels may put you at the same risk of having a stroke as if you had a pack-a-day cigarette habit.

Since then, a lot of good work has been done connecting homocysteine and coronary heart disease, mostly by M. Rene Malinow, M.D., of Oregon, and the results are important for your cardiac health: Homocysteine levels do seem to correlate to a higher risk of heart disease. One study showed that high homocysteine levels led to a three-time increase in the likelihood of stroke among young women—the same as smoking a pack of cigarettes a day.

And it appears to be more than a marker. Homocysteine is an abrasive that irritates the inside of the arteries, making them more susceptible to penetration by LDL. It also appears to stimulate smooth muscle production, which contributes to growth of plaque. It makes it easier for LDL to move into the arterial walls and may also play a role in platelet stickiness and blood clotting.

To treat or not to treat?

What we don't necessarily know is whether or not treating high homocysteine reduces your risk of coronary heart disease. There have been many studies connecting high levels of homocysteine and coronary artery disease, but there has been no major study done on what happens when we lower it. Some of these studies are in progress as I write this, so stay tuned.

That said, studies have proven that lowering blood homocysteine improves overall vascular health by promoting the relaxation of artery walls, making them less likely to spasm. It prevents **restenosis**, which means it decreases the chance that an artery that has already been surgically repaired with a stent or through angioplasty will become blocked again. A study in Switzerland demonstrated that when patients took folic acid and B vitamins, which lower homocysteine levels, after their angioplasties, they were less likely to clog up in 6 months than patients who didn't take them.

If that is not enough, I collaborated with Dr. Malinow and Dr. Spencer King of Atlanta to study different blood homocysteine levels as they relate to death in heart patients. In this study, blood homocysteine levels less than 10 μmol/L were associated with a death rate of 9 percent as compared to a death rate of 26 percent to 35 percent in those with homocysteine values more than 10 μmol/L.

As far as I'm concerned, there are lots of reasons to err on the side of caution and treat high homocysteine levels when we see them in cardiac patients. I believe that lowering homocysteine lowers risk of coronary heart disease. Since the treatment has few side effects and is inexpensive, I always opt to treat patients who have a high risk for heart disease and show elevated homocysteine.

Popeye Was Right

This is how spinach, which is rich in B vitamins, can save your life: The therapy for elevated homocysteine is to take B vitamins, including B_6, B_{12}, and folic acid. An **enzyme** is a protein that takes two chemicals, puts them together, and facilitates a reaction between them; a **cofactor** is a chemical that speeds that process up. B vitamins are the cofactors for the enzymes that get rid of homocysteine. If you have a deficiency of the enzyme that clears homocysteine from the bloodstream, B vitamins can bring the process back to normal.

We'll discuss B vitamin supplements in greater detail in the Supplement Prescription chapter, but a word of warning is appropriate here: You *must* talk to your doctor before taking any kind of supplement, especially the Bs. Folic acid in high doses requires a prescription and may block the diagnosis of a blood condition called pernicious anemia, and high doses of B_6 can cause permanent nerve damage. Supplementation should be strictly monitored by a medical professional.

If you have high homocysteine and there are no contraindications, your physician will probably put you on B vitamins in the form of supplements, but a diet rich in green, B-rich vegetables like spinach can prevent you from getting in trouble in the first place. Here's a good example: Levels of homocysteine tend to be high among the elderly, and we initially thought that as with most other things, the homocysteine-clearing enzyme was working more slowly and inefficiently in older people. This may be true, but the real culprit is the diet of the elderly, which tends to be restricted and is less likely to include the leafy green vegetables that are high in folic acid and B vitamins. When their diets are supplemented with B vitamin–rich foods, the problem tends to correct itself.

Since you don't eat homocysteine, you can't avoid it, but you can avoid eating its precursor, an amino acid called methionine. Methionine is mostly found in animal proteins, like chicken, pork, and beef, so it's best to avoid those foods and choose vegetarian proteins like soy products instead. You can also deliberately choose to increase the B vitamins in your diet by eating more fruit and leafy green vegetables—good advice in any case.

This homocysteine issue is a good example of the way that physicians weigh potential benefits of a treatment against the risks. If we discover in 5 years that lowering homocysteine is totally ineffective at preventing coronary heart disease, the cost to my patients—both financially and physically—has been negligible; they've taken some extra B vitamins. If the treatment were toxic or even slightly dangerous, we wouldn't do it. But there's very strong science to support the decisions to treat this condition, and with such terrific potential benefit and very little downside, I treat high homocysteine when I see it.

Lipoprotein (a): Stealth Heart Attack Radar
Abnormal result: 20 milligrams per deciliter (mg/dl) or above

A high level of lipoprotein (a), also known as Lp(a) (pronounced "lp little a"), is another serious independent indicator of risk for coronary artery disease. High levels of Lp(a) are present in one-third of all coronary patients, and 15 to 30 percent of people who experience premature cardiac events have elevated Lp(a).

It's another independent marker: High levels of Lp(a) raise your risk of coronary artery disease 300 percent, even if all your other numbers look good. It's hereditary, and it doesn't appear to be influenced by the lifestyle factors that many of these other markers respond to. It has been described as a "rogue gene" since it always seems to be firing and doesn't seem to be much affected by environment.

In other words, the presence of Lp(a) may be one of the reasons for the "I can't believe he had a heart attack!

> **High levels of Lp(a) are present in one-third of all coronary patients. This marker raises your risk of coronary artery disease by 300 percent.**

His cholesterol numbers/blood pressure/diet/exercise habits were fabulous!" syndrome. Lp(a) is also a dramatic risk multiplier, which means it's most dangerous in combination with another risk factor, like high LDL cholesterol. It's an equal threat to men and women, although estrogen inhibits it at the DNA level.

Lp(a) is well-known and easily recognizable, but it's undetectable unless you look for it. Since a screen for it isn't included in most routine blood work, most people don't know they have it.

When Healing Hurts

Lp(a) is an LDL particle manufactured in the liver, with an abnormal protein, called **protein (a)**, attached to it. Lp(a) isn't inherently bad: One of its functions may be to aid with healing arterial wounds. As we've discussed before, inflammation is a normal healing process; but problems start when the injury takes place in the artery and the injury is chronic. Lp(a) also encourages the growth of smooth muscle, another function of healing. All this is fine and dandy until you're doing chronic damage to the arteries with something like a high-fat diet or a cigarette smoking habit. Then the wound healing goes into overdrive, which encourages the growth of plaque that can eventually block the entire artery. Lp(a) is also susceptible to nasty oxidative damage, and once Lp(a) is oxidized, the white blood cells responsible for cleaning up the arteries gobble it up 60 times faster than normal, which makes oxidation and Lp(a) a hot topic in current medical research.

While it can be very helpful to know your Lp(a) values, there's still no standard that clinical labs can compare their values to, and consequently, commercial Lp(a) values may be inaccurate. One investigation we conducted at the Berkeley HeartLab indicated a huge difference in Lp(a) values reported by three commercial labs compared to our own research-quality test. If you want to get accurate Lp(a) values, you'd do best to get them measured in a research lab that shares quality control samples with other research laboratories. In this way, you can compare your Lp(a) value with those published in the medical journals.

Treating Lp(a)

As we've noted, lifestyle changes—diet and exercise—don't seem to affect Lp(a), and the popular cholesterol-lowering statin drugs don't have an effect, either. I'm concerned if I see Lp(a) over 20 mg/dl and prefer to see it even lower, around 15 mg/dl.

There are two practical drug treatments to lower Lp(a). It has been known for many years that estrogen can reduce Lp(a), and in a recent federal study of hormone therapy (HT) and heart disease, cardiovascular events were significantly reduced in the 25 percent of postmenopausal women who had lowered their elevated Lp(a) with HT. Obviously, this is only a solution for women, and it's a controversial one. Nicotinic acid, or niacin, also lowers Lp(a) and is the drug we use most often to do so. There are other, emerging ways to deal with this problem, but these are still too new to be entirely practical.

If we discover that you have high levels of Lp(a), it drives us to be much more aggressive about your other metabolic disorders, ones that are more responsive to the treatment options we have available to us.

Apolipoprotein E: The Diet Responder
Abnormal results: gene type E2 or E4

Like apo B, apo E is a protein attached to some lipoprotein particles. The kind of apo E you carry provides a lot of information about your risk level and how responsive you'll be to certain kinds of treatment.

I know this looks a little complicated, but stay with it: The apo E gene has three major types—E2, E3, and E4—and since you inherit one from each parent, everyone has a combination of two types. There are six general combinations possible: E2/2, E3/2, E3/3, E4/2, E4/3, and E4/4. Anything to do with 2 and 4 is a genetic mutation, or abnormality. The most common allele, or gene type, is E3—so if both your apo E alleles are E3, we call that E3/3. If you have one E3 and one E4, that's E4/3. If you have one E3 and one E2, you're an E3/2.

It's worth it to find out which E you are: E4s (which is to say, any of the combinations that include a 4) are at a substantially higher risk for heart disease.

If You're Apo E, Your Numbers Are What You Eat

The best thing about apo E is that it tells us who will respond well to a diet program in order to reduce LDL-C. If you are E2/2, you have the potential to develop **type 3 hyperlipidemia**, a classic lipid disorder characterized by deposits called **tuberoeruptive xanthoma**, which are even less attractive than they sound: marbles of fat under your skin that often occur around the elbows and the eyes and on the back. Unfortunately, these marbles also occur in the coronary arteries, which is part of the reason that people with type 3 hyperlipidemia are at a two- or threefold higher risk for coronary artery disease. Those with type 3 hyperlipidemia do best on a low-calorie, controlled-sugar diet. If they eat sugar, their problem goes crazy.

Here's an interesting fact: Only 5 percent of E2/2s have this type 3 hyperlipidemia. The rest of them are genetically predisposed, but they've ducked the gun and kept the problem under control by maintaining a healthy weight. This is a *perfect* illustration of a gene-environment interaction: an inherited condition that can be controlled completely through healthy lifestyle choices. Your genes aren't your destiny—as in so many cases, through a sensible weight management and exercise program, you can cut them off at the pass. If this condition does develop, we can usually control it with niacin and fibrates—and a low-fat, low-sugar diet.

E2 is fairly rare, but E4s (either E4/3s or E4/4s) account for between 20 and 25 percent of the healthy U.S. population. They're at higher risk for coronary heart disease, but like pattern B people, their condition is very responsive to treatment. Like E2s, E4s are real diet responders. If they eat a diet rich in fat and cholesterol, their LDL cholesterol skyrockets. If they eat a diet low in fat and cholesterol, it plummets. This makes them easier to treat: Often no drugs are necessary to correct an elevated LDL-C, and we can get great results. But if they pig out for any period of time, they're in real trouble, and their LDL-C can increase more than you'd expect.

One study shows how responsive E4s can be to diet: A group of subjects with known E types were put on diets to control their LDL cholesterol. The E3s went down a respectable 14 percent—a significant amount. The E2s similarly saw a 16 percent reduction in small LDL. But the E4s went down a more dramatic 23 percent. This goes to show how much difference the right diet can make.

An Alzheimer's predictor?

One of the problems that has cropped up with testing for apo E is that the presence of E4 seems to be connected to a risk of developing Alzheimer's disease. In 1993, *Science* magazine published the results of a study showing that in people with a family history of Alzheimer's, there was a significant correlation between apo E alleles and the chances of developing the disease. If you're an E3/3, you have approximately a 20 percent risk compared with the population at large. With E4/3, your risk goes up to 49 percent, and with E4/4, the risk is as high as 90 percent.

This raises thorny ethical questions, and it's important to note that the American Society of Human Genetics recommends that the test *not* be used to predict Alzheimer's disease risk. There are too many complications involved. First of all, there's the issue of patient reaction. Someone came to see me after reading about the test in the *Wall Street Journal*. Before we took her blood, I asked her why she wanted the test. She said, "My mother died of Alzheimer's, and if I'm in a high-risk bracket, I'm going to sell everything I own and travel the world while I can still enjoy it." Obviously, that's not a responsible reaction—if you have a 50 percent chance of getting Alzheimer's, you also have a 50 percent chance of not getting it. After some careful conversation, she agreed to talk to a counselor before taking the test.

Another patient, someone I had already been seeing, read about the Alzheimer's connection and asked me for the test. It wasn't appropriate in his case and I told him so, but I asked why he wanted it. His father had died recently, and the cost of long-term care had practically bankrupted the surviving family. He wanted to know if his risk was high so that he could purchase long-term-care insurance in preparation. I tell these two stories to demonstrate how complex this situation is.

There's another ethical dilemma for doctors and patients involved with this test. Let's say you have it done because your cardiologist needs the results to make informed decisions about your heart health care, and he puts the results in your chart. If an insurance company paid for the test, they'd have the right to that information—and all that it implies. If they knew you have a 95 percent chance of developing Alzheimer's, would they deny you insurability? In other words, is a genetic predisposition a preexisting condition? There's legislature under discussion to prevent this kind of insurance denial, but you can see how tricky it gets.

Here's what I do with my patients in the clinic. I tell them that there's a test that can help me to guide them to certain diet programs, but that the test may also give us information about their risk for Alzheimer's if there's a history of the disease in their family. If there is no history of Alzheimer's in the family, we really don't know what implications the E4 information has for Alzheimer's disease risk. If there is a family history, I ask them if they're sure they want the information. Sometimes they say no, and we just forget about doing the test at all, which is fine; apo E isn't the only way to tell if someone's a diet responder. If they say yes, I tell them that if the insurance company pays for the test, then the company has the right to have access to the results. Many patients opt to pay for the test themselves.

ADVANCED METABOLIC MARKER PROFILE: SELF-ASSESSMENT QUIZ #2

ONCE YOU'VE TAKEN THE ADVANCED METABOLIC MARKER screening tests and have gotten your results back, you'll be ready to complete your Cardiac Fingerprint. And that means you're finally in a position to know the answer to that all-important question: *What's your personal risk for coronary heart disease or a heart attack?*

Note: We're assuming that your HDL and LDL subclasses were measured using a process called gradient gel electrophoresis. This is the technique used in the National Institutes of Health–funded studies that were used as the research basis for this book. You should know that other methods of obtaining these measurements are considered to be less accurate.

To complete your profile, enter the number that corresponds with the answer you chose on the line provided.

1. LDL size (this is the diameter of the most prominent LDL particles, recorded in angstroms)

≤ 257 angstroms   6

258–262 angstroms   2

≥ 263 angstroms   0

Your LDL size score: _____

2. Do you have more than one type of LDL, and is one small?

Yes   1

No   0

Your LDL type score: _____

■ *Note: Look for two or more peaks on your lab results, much like the twin peaks of a mountain range.*

3. What is your apo B result?

> 110 mg/dl   4

80–110 mg/dl   0

< 80 mg/dl   -2

Your apo B score: _____

4. What is your HDL2b result? (postmenopausal female not on hormone therapy = male)

Male

≤ 10%   4

11–20%   3

21–30%   1

31–40%   0

> 40%   -3

Female

≤ 20%   4

21–30%   2

31–35%   1

36–40%   0

> 40%   -2

Your HDL2b score: _____

5. What is your high-sensitivity C-reactive protein (hs-CRP) score?

0–0.2 mg/dl   0

0.3–0.4 mg/dl   1

> 0.4 mg/dl   3

Your hs-CRP score: _____

6. What is your fibrinogen result?

< 400 mg/dl   0

≥ 400 mg/dl   2

Don't know   0

Your fibrinogen score: _____

7. Have you tested positive for *Chlamydia pneumoniae*?

Yes   1

No   0

Don't know   0

Your *Chlamydia pneumoniae* score: _____

8. What is your insulin result?

> 12 mU/ml   4

10–12 mU/ml   0

< 10 mU/ml   -1

Your insulin score: _____

9. What is your homocysteine result?

≤ 10 μmol/L   0

11–14 μmol/L   2

> 14 μmol/L   3

Your homocysteine score: _____

10. What is your lipoprotein (a) (Lp[a]) result?

≤ 20 mg/dl   0

21–25 mg/dl   1

26–30 mg/dl   2

> 30 mg/dl   3

Your Lp(a) score: _____

11. Do you have the apo E4 allele?

Yes   2

No   0

Don't know   0

Your apo E4 score: _____

■ *Note: On your report, this will appear as E4/3 or E4/4.*

12. Are you apo E type 2/2?

Yes   2

No   0

Don't know   0

Your apo E2/2 score: _____

■ *Note: On your report, this will appear as E2/2. An E3/2 does not count.*

13. What's your LDL-C result?

≤ 80 mg/dl   -3

81–99 mg/dl   -1

100–129 mg/dl   1

130–160 mg/dl   3

> 160 mg/dl   5

Your LDL-C score: _____

14. Do you have a history of LDL-C over 130 that you've now brought down to less than 100 mg/dl?

Yes   -1

No   0

Your LDL-C reduction score: _____

15. What is your HDL-C result? (postmenopausal female not on hormone therapy = male)

	Male	Female
≤ 40 mg/dl	4	6
41–45 mg/dl	1	6
46–50 mg/dl	0	4
51–55 mg/dl	-1	1
56–60 mg/dl	-3	0
61–65 mg/dl	-3	-1
≥ 66 mg/dl	-4	-3

Your HDL-C history score: _____

(continued)

ADVANCED METABOLIC MARKER PROFILE: SELF-ASSESSMENT QUIZ #2 (*cont.*)

16. Do you have a history of low HDL-C that you've brought up to above 50 mg/dl (in men or postmenopausal women) or above 60 (in pre-menopausal women or women on hormone therapy)?

Yes   -2

No   0

Your HDL-C increase score: _____

17. What is your triglyceride result?

≥ 150 mg/dl   3

100–149 mg/dl   1

70–99 mg/dl   0

< 70 mg/dl   -2

Your fasting triglyceride score: _____

Your total Advanced Metabolic Marker Profile score: _____

Our next step is to use this score, combined with your score from the Personal Risk Profile in chapter 3, to determine your relative risk of heart disease and cardiac event. We'll call this final score your Cardiac Fingerprint score.

A number-oriented tunnel vision severely limits our ability to accurately assess your risk and treat your conditions. All of us are different. When we take your whole Cardiac Fingerprint into account, we find that a whole new world opens up. We know in precise terms what you're up against and, most important, how to help customize a treatment approach for you.

We'll now combine your Personal Risk Profile score with your Advanced Metabolic Marker score to come up with your Cardiac Fingerprint score.

First, take your score from the Personal Risk Profile on page 38. Depending on your score, you'll be assigned a number: your "risk multiplier."

If your score is a negative number or zero, your multiplier is × 1.
If your score is between 1 and 3, your risk multiplier is × 1.
If your score is between 4 and 6, your risk multiplier is × 2.
If your score is between 7 and 10, your risk multiplier is × 3.
If your score is 11 or above, your risk multiplier is × 4.

The next step is to multiply your Advanced Metabolic Marker score by your risk multiplier. This will give you your Cardiac Fingerprint score.

Your Cardiac Fingerprint score is the number that really counts. It's what tells you and your doctor with greater certainty how likely you are to develop heart disease or to experience a cardiac event. Of course, no risk prediction tool is perfect, but you will find a real profusion of information here, compared to what you're used to.

Let's go through an example together.

Joe's score on the Personal Risk Profile was an 11. That gives him the highest risk multiplier possible, × 4. His score from the Advanced Metabolic Marker Profile was a 19. To determine his true Cardiac Fingerprint, he now multiplies his score of 19 by 4, (19 × 4) to reach 76. If you take a look at "Your Cardiac Scorecard" below along with Joe, you'll see that he measures at the outer extreme for risk of coronary heart disease.

Your risk multiplier × Your score from Advanced Metabolic Marker Profile
= Your Cardiac Fingerprint score = Your true risk assessment

YOUR CARDIAC SCORECARD

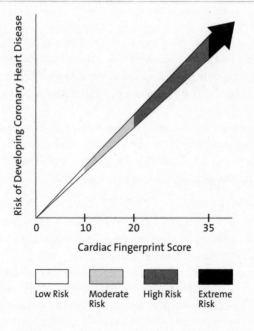

(continued)

ADVANCED METABOLIC MARKER PROFILE: UNDERSTANDING YOUR CARDIAC SCORECARD

0–10: Low Risk

Your risk of heart attack is extremely low. Keep up the good work! Stay alert to changes in your medical status and have regular checkups with your physician.

11–20: Moderate Risk

You're definitely at elevated risk for coronary heart disease; you have sufficient metabolic abnormalities to suggest that you're in the risk zone. Don't despair! Your Cardiac Fingerprint allows you and your doctor to take control of your cardiac destiny. I recommend that you and your physician begin at once to treat your underlying metabolic disorder(s) and address any poor lifestyle issues.

After you've gotten started on the individualized plans that will put you on the road to a healthier heart, I recommend you go back for physician review and retesting in 3 months. This allows you and your doctor to adjust your plan accordingly.

21–34: High Risk

You are at high risk for developing coronary heart disease or suffering some form of cardiac event (but that's only if you don't take action!) If you score in this range, you and your physician need to make serious adjustments to your lifestyle right away, and your doctor may want also to think about medication for you (at least for the short term).

If one or more of these abnormal markers indicate that you might be in immediate danger, then medication is the best first step. Your primary care physician may refer you to a specialist in metabolic cardiology. Then you can begin to build a heart health plan that comprises diet, exercise, and supplements.

35 + Extreme Risk

You're at *extremely high risk* of a cardiac event. Make a doctor's appointment tomorrow, and prepare to make radical changes in your lifestyle. It is probable that your physician will want to start you on medication.

Next, get ready to take charge of your cardiac destiny. By embarking on the right diet and exercise plans, you will be able not only to control, but in many instances, actually correct the underlying metabolic conditions that put you at risk in the first place.

THE LIGHT AT THE END OF THE TUNNEL

As you can now see, if we can get away from our cholesterol-dominated tunnel vision, we find ourselves with a much more realistic—and much more effective—approach to recognizing and treating the root causes of coronary heart disease.

Clearly, these additional diagnostic markers provide us with the information that can make all the difference when choosing treatment options. And all this lifesaving data comes from nothing more complicated than a blood test! Once you've seen the light, it gets harder and harder to understand why these screening tests aren't being recommended for patients in every cardiologist's office throughout the country.

In the next chapter, we'll talk about how you can arrange to be tested: how to introduce the topic with your doctor, where to get tested, who pays for it, and how to interpret your results.

5

GETTING TESTED

IN THE LAST CHAPTER, you got a glimpse of what we can learn from new tests for metabolic and inherited disorders that affect your heart. Our ability to identify these new and specific markers has propelled cardiology to a new level in terms of preventing, detecting, and treating coronary heart disease.

Hopefully, the information in the last chapter, combined with your own results from the Personal Risk Profile, has convinced you that there's valuable information to be gathered from these extra metabolic marker tests. You're no doubt eager to take the next step.

But how will you go about getting these tests? Do you need to have special connections? Will your doctor even know what you're talking about? Who will pay for them? What do you actually need to do? And how do you read the results once you get your lab report back? I know from dealing with my own patients how many practical, logistical questions you must have at this point, and in this chapter, I'm going to do my best to answer them. Whether you're trying to decide how to approach your busy doctor or trying to decode your lab results, this section is devoted to helping you get on with the process of dealing with your heart.

It always takes a little time for any new science to filter down from the researchers to the doctors to their patients. My intention is to close that research gap so that you can benefit from this revolution in diagnostics today.

TALKING TO YOUR DOCTOR

We're all different. We're metabolically different, we have different medical histories, and we have different levels of commitment to our health. It's unrealistic to expect that we'll all respond similarly to treatments. I believe that the mark of a good physician is the ability to look at all of the scientific "ingredients" that make up a patient, throw in a little information about risk and lifestyle, and come up with a personalized path of therapy designed specifically to meet the needs of the individual patient.

That said, the way medicine is paid for these days discourages individualized treatment. Much attention is paid to what's cost-effective, which in my opinion has more to do with what's best for the financial health of the insurance company footing the bill and less to do with what's best for the patient. Individualized treatment takes a lot of the physician's time, and spending a long time with a single patient is often discouraged because it means that he can see fewer of them. As a result, the brunt of the responsibility for preventive medicine often falls on the patient. This is one reason for this book.

It seems that health care is divided into two tiers these days. If you're really wealthy, you can walk into your doctor's office on Fifth Avenue and he or she will order a whole battery of tests, cost no object. You'll probably leave with an accurate risk profile and an appropriate therapy path—but what about people who can't afford that kind of treatment? Another tier is beginning to emerge—people who do their homework and insist on participating actively in choices about their health care. You don't have to be superwealthy to get terrific medical care: You just have to educate yourself and then find a medical professional who encourages your interaction on decisions about your care.

I know that sometimes people find it difficult to communicate with their doctors. You don't want to seem critical or paranoid or neurotic by asking for a whole bunch of tests he or she hasn't already determined necessary. And sometimes their responses can be harder to decipher than their handwriting.

So how should you broach the subject of these advanced tests? First of all, you need to know that there's nothing wrong with taking information to your physician. My patients bring me clippings from mainstream newspapers and even from medical journals all the time, and sometimes they contain very helpful information that I wouldn't have had access to without their intervention. Even if it's something I'm already aware of, I'm happy to answer questions and talk about why I've chosen one treatment over another. A well-educated patient is an asset to my practice, and I'm always pleased when my patients take an active role in their own health care and treatment.

There's so much new science being reported these days that it's almost impossible to keep up, so your doctor may very well not yet be familiar with this science. You have every right to bring it to his attention. But tone is everything. If you give your doctor this information in a way that implies you've caught him napping on the job or trying to deny you the best care possible, he's going to get defensive. I'd suggest that you take some documentation when you go. (This book should do nicely.) Ask him what he thinks of testing for these additional markers and whether or not he thinks you're a good candidate for these tests. Listen carefully to what he says. If you've read this book and you believe that you are a good candidate, you'll have more than enough information to make a coherent argument for additional tests. (At the back of this book, I have also included references to articles in well-respected medical journals for those physicians who would like to learn more.)

If your doctor recommends that you not do the tests but you wish to do them anyway, you're within your rights to explain your feelings and ask that he arrange to have them done. You can also ask him to put you in touch with a cardiologist who can give you a second opinion and who will do the testing for you, if you meet the necessary medical criteria. Obtaining a second opinion is a time-honored tradition in medicine and one that you should exercise without hesitation when you have doubts. If you or your physician needs to find a doctor who specializes in **lipid metabolism**, which involves the Advanced Metabolic Markers, Berkeley HeartLab (patient hotline: 866-871-4408, toll-free, Pacific Standard Time), the laboratory I helped to found through the University of California, Berkeley, will provide you with names of doctors in your area who are familiar with these tests.

WHERE THE TESTS ARE DONE

When you and your doctor have agreed that these tests are the logical next step, he will take blood from you and send it out to a specialized lab for analysis. There are a number of laboratories that can test for these additional markers.

Obviously, all my lab work goes to Berkeley HeartLab. When we started the lab, we were one of the few places in the country doing this work. Thankfully, the word has spread. Be aware that many of these advanced tests don't have a national standard, so it's up to your physician to determine if the lab is doing the tests accurately. Unfortunately, it's not a given, so your doctor will need to choose carefully.

Whichever lab you end up choosing will have special requirements for the way the blood should be drawn and shipped to it. Your doctor's office will have that information.

PREPARING FOR THE TEST

Your doctor will give you a set of specific instructions so you know exactly what to do before you take the test, but here's a glimpse of what you can expect.

Do you need to fast?

You'll need to fast for 12 to 14 hours prior to the blood draw for the test. You may drink water, but you should not consume any alcohol for 24 hours before the blood draw.

FINDING A RELIABLE LABORATORY

Finding a reliable laboratory isn't always easy. Your doctor will most likely have experience with a number of labs and can address your concerns if you have them. Here are some indicators that your doctor can use to determine the level of quality control at a laboratory.

DOES THE LAB PARTICIPATE IN MAJOR NATIONAL RESEARCH STUDIES?
One way to ensure that the lab is accurate is to find one that participates in big research studies, which means there's always some kind of external oversight process and quality control is of utmost importance.

IS THE LAB LINKED TO NATIONAL STANDARDS?
The government sells samples of total cholesterol that are guaranteed to be reliable measures. This is a good way for a lab to test its machines—if a machine gives a value of 84 and the government has guaranteed that the sample has a value of 100, then the lab knows something's wrong with its machine.

There is national standardization for the more common tests, such as total cholesterol and triglycerides. There is none for the more esoteric tests, though, which is one of the reasons it's important to use a reliable lab: Labs involved in research often share their own standardization samples. Someone could set up a facility to test for Lp(a), for example, but if it doesn't have any standard to calibrate its machine to, then you won't be able to relate your result to any of the numbers published in major medical research studies.

This is called a fasting blood test. Don't cheat! If you've eaten in the hours prior to having your blood drawn, it can affect your blood lipid level, especially your triglycerides.

What if you're already taking medication for your heart?
If you're already on lipid metabolism medication (statins, beta-blockers, niacin, fibrates, etc.), you should ask your doctor whether he'd like you to stop taking these drugs before you're tested. It's best to be tested without med-

DOES THE LAB SAVE THE BLOOD SAMPLE FOR 1 TO 2 WEEKS IN CASE OF A PROBLEM? WILL IT RERUN THE TEST IF THE RESULT SEEMS ABNORMAL, AND WILL IT DO THAT FOR FREE?

It's not unusual for a doctor to get a test result back that doesn't look the way he was expecting it to. A good lab will keep the sample for a week or two in a refrigerator so that if there's any doubt, it can run the numbers again. A willingness to retest a sample—and to do it for free—is a good indicator of a lab's commitment to quality control.

WHAT'S THE COEFFICIENT OF VARIATION ON A PARTICULAR TEST?

This is the amount that the lab's results vary around an absolute known value. Your doctor can call and speak to a lab's director, and he'll have this information. For cholesterol measurements, it should be less than 3 percent (and in a good research lab, less than 1 percent).

DOES IT USE A PROCESS CALLED GRADIENT GEL ELECTROPHORESIS TO DETERMINE THE 5-HDL AND 7-LDL SUBCLASSES?

That's the technique used in the National Institutes of Health–funded studies upon which the research for this book is based. The "gold standard" is a method called analytic ultracentrifugation (ANUC), but it is cumbersome and very expensive. However, the gradient gel electrophoresis method I use is calibrated to ANUC. Other measurement methods are not as reliable. **I highly recommend that physicians choose only those labs that use this technique.**

ication so we're sure the drugs aren't masking a condition that would otherwise alert us to test your family members for the same condition.

If you and your physician decide that you will go off the drugs in order to be tested, we suggest that you discontinue the drug for a minimum of 4 weeks prior to the test (6 to 8 weeks is ideal). Obviously, if stopping the drug would compromise your health, you should be tested while on the drug. Do not stop any medications without first talking to your physician.

What about your other medications?

Other medications you may be taking for totally unrelated problems (like your arthritis) may make your blood tests look better or worse. This is why your doctor should have a full list of all the medications you're taking. He'll be able to tell you whether it's best for you to go off the other medication for a period of time before you're tested. Whether you do or not, he'll be able to take the effects of those other medications into account when reviewing your results.

MAKING SENSE OF YOUR LAB RESULTS

You'll refer to your numbers for various purposes throughout this book, so I thought it would be useful to provide you with a separate, easy-to-read chart where you can "store" the relevant numbers for easy access instead of having to consult the lab report every time you need to know what your metabolic marker levels are.

Since the whole point of this book is to help you to improve your numbers, I'd encourage you to fill in your results on the opposite page. I'm confident that your numbers are going to change for the better, so make a few photocopies of this page, and fill in a new chart every time you get retested. Date the top of each one, and you'll have a permanent record of your improvement.

Let's transfer your lab result scores together into the Quick Reference Chart. You'll find, for example, that the first item on the list is total cholesterol, at the top of the left-hand column. Now, refer to your own lab report to find the results of your total cholesterol and place that number into the Your Result column. Notice that in the Abnormal Levels column I've also provided you with a cutoff number that enables you immediately to see whether your results are normal or abnormal. If your result is higher or lower than the cutoff number provided in this column, that means your result is abnormal, and you'll put a "yes" in the Abnormal Result column. If your result is normal, you'll put a "no" in that column.

QUICK REFERENCE CHART: Your Cardiac Stats

Date:

Metabolic Markers	Abnormal Levels	Your Result	Abnormal Result?
Standard lipid panel			
Total cholesterol (mg/dl)	≥ 200		
LDL-C (mg/dl)	≥ 130		
HDL-C (mg/dl):			
Premenopausal women and women on hormone therapy	≤ 50		
Men and postmenopausal women	≤ 40		
Triglycerides (mg/dl)	≥ 140		
Additional markers			
HDL2b (% total cholesterol):			
Premenopausal women and women on hormone therapy	$\leq 35\%$		
Men and postmenopausal women	$\leq 20\%$		
LDL size, peak #1 (pattern B; angstroms) or LDL IIIa + IIIb	≤ 257 $\geq 20\%$		
Apolipoprotein B (mg/dl)	≥ 80		
High-sensitivity C-reactive protein (mg/dl)	≥ 0.4		
Fibrinogen (mg/dl)	≥ 400		
Chlamydia pneumoniae	$\geq 1{:}32$		
Insulin (mU/ml)	≥ 12		
Homocysteine (μmol/L)	≥ 14		
Lipoprotein (a) (mg/dl)	≥ 20		
Apolipoprotein E	*E4, E2 gene types*		

Note: The numbers we are using here are considerably lower that those traditionally used to define "abnormal" in medicine. When we use the term here, it is simply meant to indicate that your result places you at higher-than-average risk—but not in the grossly inflated range that the term "abnormal" ordinarily connotes in medicine.

So, returning to total cholesterol, if the cutoff number is 200, and your test results are in fact greater than or equal to (≥) 200 mg/dl, then your results are abnormal and you'd enter "yes" in the last column. Do the same for LDL-C, HDL-C, going down the list, inserting "yes" or "no" in that last column according to your own results. (If your lab report includes its own cutoff numbers, you may see some discrepancies here. These are the cutoff numbers that I use in my own practice, based on my own research and that of others in the field; I believe that these numbers are the most helpful.)

So the first line of your results might look like this.

Metabolic Markers	Abnormal Levels	Your Result	Abnormal Result?
Standard lipid panel			
Total cholesterol (mg/dl)	≥ 200	275	Yes

Each Nutrition, Exercise, Supplement, and Medication Prescription requires that you know which of your results is abnormal so that you can determine which program is right for you. You'll be referring back to this page later on when you work your way through the Prescription section of the book in part 2.

I want you to be able to access the information you'll need at a single glance, so after you've finished filling out the chart, take one more step to get rid of all the numbers. You can further simplify the chart by cutting out every column except the Abnormal Result column. All you need to do is place a "yes" in the column next to each item for which you listed "yes" in the above chart (or a "no" if your result is normal).

Metabolic Markers	Abnormal Result?
Standard lipid panel	
Total cholesterol	
LDL-C	
HDL-C	
Triglycerides	
Additional markers	
HDL2b	
LDL pattern B	
Apolipoprotein B	
High-sensitivity C-reactive protein	
Fibrinogen	
Chlamydia pneumoniae	
Insulin	
Homocysteine	
Lipoprotein (a)	
Apolipoprotein E	

Now you have a quick and easy reference that lists all of your markers—and that's all you'll need to find your individualized plans in the Prescription section.

A NOTE ABOUT CUTOFF NUMBERS

As I've already mentioned, cutoff numbers are necessary, but I find that they can be misleading when not understood and used properly. **These numbers always need to be put into the context of the patient's unique and individual medical and family history, and that's a job for your doctor.**

For instance, studies have shown that your risk of heart attack goes up if your homocysteine is over 14. But in some people, those who already have established coronary heart disease, the threshold is lower and their risk increases significantly when homocysteine climbs above 10. So there's a substantial difference in those cutoff numbers, depending on your history. A safe level of homocysteine for one person is not necessarily a safe level for everyone in every instance.

Another example: If you have established coronary heart disease, then I'm going to be much more aggressive in my efforts to get your HDL2b, or "good cholesterol," as high as it can go—I'm going to hammer you with as much niacin as you can comfortably tolerate in an effort to stop the progression of your disease. In someone without coronary heart disease, I'd be satisfied if these numbers were within the high-normal range.

The acceptable range varies according to the patient's history, but it also varies according to the levels of the other markers. Many of these factors are especially dangerous when they're combined with one another. A triglyceride level of 140 might be normal in someone with LDL pattern A cholesterol— but that same triglyceride level indicates a greater level of danger for someone with LDL pattern B.

So depending on your history and your own constellation of risk factors, your cutoff numbers can—and should—differ from the standard. We all have to work for *our own best numbers*, and that means taking a wide range of factors into account—and the more information we have, the more factors we need to consider.

I'd also like to remind you again that these cutoff numbers aren't written in stone. If the cutoff is 100, and you're at 98, you're not in the clear! Risk doesn't drop precipitously on the other side of that cutoff number.

I don't mean to negate the validity of cutoff numbers altogether. They provide valuable and essential guidelines; without standards, we would be lost. But you now see why some of my numbers are more conservative than you might be accustomed to; I'd rather have you reach for the best numbers possible than settle complacently at a number that might still put you at risk. And I would encourage you, going forward, to think of all cutoff numbers as the center of a range rather than the edge of a cliff.

This is why it is so important for you to have open communication and a solid working partnership with your doctor. Consider these numbers guidelines, and review them with your physician in the context of your medical history.

INSURANCE COVERAGE

You're probably wondering, who's going to pay for these tests? The answer is: It depends.

In most cases, it's the difference between primary and secondary care. If you have no evidence of coronary heart disease at all and no evidence of other medical problems such as diabetes, high blood pressure, or high blood fats, these tests count as primary, or preventive, care because there's "nothing wrong with you." As you probably know, preventive care is largely in the hands of the patients in this country. If you and your doctor consider you to be at high risk because of your family history, you may decide to pay for the testing yourself. The full battery costs between $400 and $600, which is not insignificant but might turn out to be the best investment you ever made.

This is a sobering story: I was fighting with one of the insurance companies a couple of years ago to get them to cover these tests. I had run the numbers based on a study I'd conducted in Texas and could prove to them that it would save them money in the long run—after 2 years, in fact, about $4,000 per cardiac patient per year. One of their representatives told me point-blank that it would never happen. Why? He said they'd never reap the rewards of that kind of preventive care. The average length of time that people stay with one insurance company is about 18 months. Either their company changes plans or the patient gets dissatisfied with the treatment he's receiving and goes to one of the other plans his workplace offers. This company's refusal to cover the tests was a business decision: They weren't going to pay for something that would end up benefiting someone else's bottom line, even if it meant the difference between health and a cardiac event for a patient. In this case, cost-effective meant choosing the financial health of the insurance company over the health of the patient.

In contrast, and on a much brighter note, I went to Medicare in California in 1999 and showed them our findings and those of other international researchers. I told them that the abundance of excellent studies indicated that patients with certain medical problems would benefit if physicians had access to these tests. They said they'd pay for the tests if we could prove three things: that the tests give physicians results that no other test does; that the results of the test led to a clear path of therapy (in other words, that Results A pointed to Diet A and Medication A); and that there was a demonstrable benefit to the patient when that treatment path was taken. We were able to demonstrate all three things with published scientific studies, they published the results in their bulletin, and many of these tests are now paid for by Medicare if the patient has the appropriate diagnostic code. (Medicare does not pay for prevention in people with no medical diagnosis.)

One of the organizations we've worked with is Kaiser Permanente Healthcare in northern California. Forward-thinking physicians in its cardiology department in San Francisco have incorporated these tests into their medical practices for many years now. Kaiser has recently reported a significant reduction in cardiovascular disease, and the cost of cardiovascular disease in its patient population has also gone down. I am proud to say that I played a part in setting up the nurse-run lipid clinics to which much of this success is attributed, through a federally funded program at Stanford University run by Robert F. DeBusk, M.D. Through aggressive prevention in the Kaiser system, cardiovascular disease rates have dropped significantly—and the system is saving a *lot* of money.

Many doctors and patients have lobbied for these tests to be covered, and many insurance companies—even HMOs—will cover at least a portion of these tests if they're included as part of secondary care. This means that if you already have coronary heart disease or a heart disease–related diagnosis, you've got a much better chance of getting your health insurance company to pay for the tests. All you need is an appropriate diagnostic code, which basically means a diagnosis for issues related to coronary heart disease risk.

The only way to tell whether you're covered for these tests is for you or your doctor's office to call your carrier directly.

PART 2

CHANGING YOUR CARDIAC DESTINY: THE PRESCRIPTIONS

6

PRESCRIPTIONS FOR LIFELONG HEART HEALTH: AN INTRODUCTION

CONGRATULATIONS! You've completed the self-assessment portion of the book, and that means it's now time to devise an action plan. In part 2, I'll walk you through the actual Prescriptions. This is where your complete Cardiac Fingerprint—that's your Personal Risk Profile score combined with the results of your Advanced Metabolic Marker tests—will point you to programs tailor-made for your cardiac profile.

If you've only completed your Personal Risk Profile and haven't yet taken the Advanced Metabolic Marker tests, that's fine. You'll still have plenty to learn in this section—and even without those advanced tests, we can still direct you to programs that will get you started on the road to a brighter cardiac future!

If you've completed both the Personal Risk Profile and the Advanced Metabolic Marker Profile, you now have a wealth of relevant information about your current heart health risk. You and your doctor can now get started without further delay on the health and lifestyle programs that can help you to change your cardiac destiny.

If you follow the programs I've formulated for your specific cardiac profile, I fully expect your metabolic marker results to change for the better. And you can (and should) start today. That's why I want you to make a note on your calendar to get retested 4 months from the day you embark on your individualized programs. I think you're going to be very pleased with the results!

It is important to retest in order to monitor how you're doing 4 months after you begin the programs and then at regular intervals to be determined with your doctor. In addition to encouraging you as your scores improve, these updates will help determine where you are making the greatest gains and also whether any areas still need adjustment.

By the way, you should also retake the Personal Risk Profile questionnaire every time you're retested. In this way, you keep updating your complete Cardiac Fingerprint and you can actually see your complete risk profile—along with your cardiac destiny—changing before your very eyes.

Note: Any time you begin a new course of treatment, you need to be monitored by your doctor. Your physician should be your partner in every new health regimen that affects your medical condition, and only your doctor can determine if you have any individual factors that would indicate you should or should not take any of the paths suggested in this book. One lesson I especially hope you take away from this book is that diet, weight loss, and exercise can be genuine therapeutic paths. That means they have the power to work tangible benefits on your cardiac health, but also that they are powerful tools that require careful oversight and monitoring by your personal physician.

So let's get started. This Cardiac Fingerprint actually answers the questions:

- What's your level of risk for coronary heart disease—or a heart attack?
- Should you and your doctor consider noninvasive tests to determine if you already have coronary heart disease?
- Should other members of your family be tested?
- What treatment plans may be most beneficial for you? And what combination of plans will enable you to control—and perhaps even reverse—the underlying metabolic imbalances that put you at risk?

WHAT'S YOUR RISK LEVEL?

As you've seen, the first thing these tests do is give us a much better indication of your risk for cardiovascular disease and heart attack. Your Cardiac Fingerprint score tells you just how high—or how low—you are on the risk gauge. So how did you rate?

Your total risk rises as the number of risk factors rises. And your overall Cardiac Fingerprint score provides us with a useful measure for how aggressive you may need to be in launching your counteroffensive.

An overweight smoker with three abnormal Advanced Metabolic Marker items had better get into gear as quickly as possible. My goal is to help people to see that they are at risk long before that first chest pain occurs. When you know that you're at risk—and know what factors are putting you there—you also gain the control you need to change your cardiac destiny.

If your scores spell serious trouble already, don't waste another minute before taking control of your cardiac future. But the lesson here is also preventive: *Everyone* needs to take stock of their cardiac status, and everyone needs to begin to take the steps necessary to ensure a heart-healthy life. Don't wait until the numbers turn or your health begins to suffer. Begin today and that day may never come!

SHOULD YOU CONSIDER NONINVASIVE TESTS?

Getting a high score on your Personal Risk Profile indicates you may get valuable information by getting the Advanced Metabolic Marker screening. If the results of those advanced screening tests indicate a number of abnormal metabolic conditions, you and your doctor will want to discuss whether it makes sense for you to undergo some noninvasive tests to determine whether you already have coronary heart disease.

The severity of the disease will obviously be another factor in determining how aggressive your treatment needs to be in order to preempt a cardiac event. Again, we must focus on obtaining as much relevant information as possible, so that you and your doctor can plan the best strategic counteroffensive. We need to know if you're already suffering any of the destructive effects of coronary heart disease to determine your treatment. The more advanced the disease, the more aggressive your treatment should be. In other words, this is all about the first strike: striking out against the disease before the heart attack strikes you.

If you and your physician do decide that some noninvasive tests are the logical next step, then he or she will explain these tests to you in greater detail. In the meantime, here's some general information about what to expect.

Electrocardiograms and Chest X-rays

Electrocardiogram (EKG), which measures changes in the electrical impulses coming from your heart, and the **chest x-ray**, which shows whether the heart is abnormally enlarged, are both good ways for your doctor to determine whether or not you already have obvious heart damage, including evidence of a previous "silent" heart attack, or an enlarged heart.

Treadmill Tests

Another very common noninvasive test is a **stress test,** which is where a doctor carefully monitors the changes in your EKG while you're doing controlled exercise, like walking or running on a treadmill. These are often called treadmill stress tests.

This test is very good at determining whether or not you have gross coronary heart disease, but it's not a particularly subtle instrument: One of your major coronary arteries has to be approximately 75 percent blocked before anything shows up on a treadmill test. Now that's pretty blocked, and plenty of people have serious cardiac incidents with a less than 75 percent blockage—in fact, most heart attacks occur because of 50 percent blockages. So treadmill tests are useful if they're positive because they'll lead you to the next step, such as a coronary arteriogram. However, a "normal" stress test does *not* mean that you do not have coronary heart disease, only that you don't have severe enough coronary heart disease to make the stress test positive. Don't be lulled into a false sense of security if your stress test is normal but your Advanced Metabolic Marker tests are not.

Treadmill tests aren't 100 percent reliable either. Lots of things can alter the electrical signals your heart sends, including salt imbalances in your blood, and even the way your heart hangs in your chest. These tests are also notoriously unreliable for premenopausal women; the electrical signals their hearts send naturally can look like disease, so the test has a high rate of false positives for women.

There are two variations on the treadmill test that can give you slightly more accurate results. The first is a **thallium exercise test**, which measures blood profusion. It's performed like a treadmill test, but instead of looking at the results of an EKG, your doctor will inject a mildly radioactive substance into your bloodstream and take pictures of your chest with what's essentially a large Geiger counter. If blood is getting everywhere it needs to go, your doctor will see a normal picture of a heart traced in radioactive dye—if there are blockages, he'll see cold spots, or black patches where the blood isn't getting through. We can detect arteries that are approximately 60 to 70 percent blocked with this test.

Another variation is the **stress echocardiogram**. You do your treadmill test, and then your doctor will bounce sound waves off your heart. Like a submarine's sonar, this test can tell us if there's some irregularity in the way your heart muscle contracts when it beats. If part of the heart is "sick" because blood isn't reaching it properly, that area will contract differently and badly, and he'll see an undulation in that spot. This test can also detect arteries that are 60 to 70 percent blocked.

Carotid Ultrasound

Another common noninvasive test we do is a carotid ultrasound. This test discovers blockages of the carotid artery in the neck, which increases stroke risk. There is a correlation between this and what's happening inside your coronary arteries: As your carotid artery wall gets thicker, the amount of coronary heart disease, as assessed by coronary arteriograms, tends to get worse as well. We'll use this test to guide therapy in patients: If your carotid artery wall thickness is stable or regressing, we know that whatever therapy we're doing is probably working in your heart arteries as well; if your carotid artery wall thickness appears to be getting worse, we'll add another drug or increase the dose of the one you're on because your heart arteries are probably getting worse.

Coronary Calcification Test

The coronary calcification test is another noninvasive test, one that measures the amount of calcium in the walls of the arteries, a signal that the body is trying to repair arterial damage. Shoe stores in the '50s used a fluoroscope to see the bones in the feet; now we use something similar to see the "bones" developing in your heart. The heart moves too fast for regular x-rays, but we now have the technology through a process called **electron beam tomography,** or **EBT,** to take multiple pictures at a very fast shutter speed and can use these to assess your calcium burden, the number of blood vessels involved, and the relative extent of the coronary heart disease. This test does not tell you how severely blocked a heart artery is, but it does tell you how much plaque burden you have. This is a good measure of the extent of coronary heart disease.

When you get your coronary calcification results, there will be two numbers: your absolute score and a percent distribution score, which compares you to other people in your gender and age category. Since calcification happens to many of us as we age, knowing how our calcium burden rates compare to those of other people in our age brackets can be very helpful. A negative calcium score in an older individual is a good sign, while a positive calcium score in a younger individual is a bad sign.

The problem, of course, as with many of these tests, is that this test doesn't really give you an idea of your risk for coronary heart disease. A low score doesn't necessarily mean that you're in the clear. The test only shows lesions that have become calcified, and in many cases, calcified lesions are more stable than ones that aren't. The calcium turns the arteries into "lead pipes"—but as we know, it's often the unstable soft plaque that can cause heart attacks. In other words, sometimes people with low calcium burdens are at higher risk of cardiac event than those with high calcium burdens. But this test is still a good indicator that your body is working to repair existing damage.

Angiogram

Another relatively common test is a **cardiac catheterization,** or coronary angiogram. This is an invasive test. Your doctor threads a thin tube up from the femoral artery in your groin into the coronary arteries and injects colored dye, which helps him to see the position and severity of the blockages in your coronary arteries on an x-ray screen. This test can tell you with a great degree of accuracy how much of a blockage you have.

Intravascular Ultrasound

The best test out there right now to assess the burden of atherosclerosis in coronary arteries is called IVUS, which stands for intravascular ultrasound. It's slightly more invasive; a coronary angiogram is performed and the catheter is threaded down one of the coronary arteries, and sound waves are bounced off the inside of the arteries, which gives us a much more accurate picture of how much atherosclerosis is actually in the wall of the artery. Remember, the disease starts in the artery wall. For many years, the artery expands to accommodate the atherosclerosis; only when the disease is well-established does it begin to narrow the *inside* of the artery. If IVUS were noninvasive, we'd do it every year on everyone with coronary heart disease to see how the disease was responding to treatment. Of course, this isn't clinically practical, although the information would be useful both to guide treatment and to determine whether or not it has been successful so far.

There is no really perfect, inexpensive, and accurate noninvasive test right now, although a number are under investigation. The ultimate goal, of course, is an accurate, inexpensive, noninvasive test that helps us do better patient management!

But here again, you'll reap the benefits of knowing the status of your Advanced Metabolic Markers. Knowing your underlying metabolic conditions greatly improves the prognostic ability of these noninvasive cardiac tests and can help your doctor to interpret the results. For instance, if you have wishy-washy results on your treadmill test (the kind that ordinarily does not send up an alarm but isn't quite normal), but your blood work looks okay, he may want you to make lifestyle changes before more serious therapies such as drugs, and then repeat the test. If your treadmill test results are suspicious without being really diagnostic, but your blood work indicates that you have a number of metabolic issues that increase your risk, he may want to be more aggressive with treatment.

SHOULD OTHER MEMBERS OF YOUR FAMILY GET TESTED?

If your Advanced Metabolic Marker results do show metabolic abnormalities, it's a good idea to see if your other primary relatives are willing to get tested as well. We cannot ever forget that these conditions often have a genetic basis, and any abnormalities in your blood work mean that those in your genetic pool are at risk from these abnormalities as well.

Your dad went on cholesterol-lowering treatment after his heart attack at age 48—don't you think his rehabilitation efforts would gain momentum if his doctor was able to treat the underlying metabolic imbalances that caused that heart attack? And knowing the results of his tests can benefit you as well. If your parents are discovered to have different metabolic imbalances from your own, that can add another layer of insight for your physician in assessing your personal data. You may be genetically inclined and simply not expressing those imbalances yet—and knowing that you're prone to them can help you make sure it stays that way.

And the next generation *really* benefits. Your healthy, athletic 29-year-old son, the one with perfectly normal results on the standard cholesterol tests? Well, if your blood work shows up with multiple genetic and metabolic abnormalities, it's more than a good idea to get his blood work done also.

Even if he's in perfect health today, it's important to know if he shares any of your predispositions. Let's say we find out he's got the same genetic and metabolic abnormalities that you and his granddad have. That's a big red flag; it indicates that your son is on the same track as the other men in your family, and we have to get him out of the way of that speeding train. So we might be more aggressive with treatment than we would in another case.

WHAT'S THE MOST BENEFICIAL TREATMENT STRATEGY FOR *YOU*?

In addition to giving you a better sense of your true level of risk, these Advanced Metabolic Marker tests also enable cardiologists to see in exquisite detail exactly where you're vulnerable and attack the problem at its source!

We don't have to wait until your arteries are actually blocked. We can see from your test results if you're going to be prone to arterial blockage, and we can fight back. In the old days, we had the weaponry, but we didn't have the advance intelligence to fight back in the early stages of arteriosclerosis, when it would have mattered most. Angioplasty and bypass surgeries were practically inevitable outcomes in

> Your Cardiac Fingerprint provides the blueprint for a customized set of treatment plans that are tailor-made for your particular metabolic needs.

many instances—if you were prone to arterial blockage, we'd see you in the operating room at some future date.

But if I told you that by making adjustments to what you ate and how you exercised, you could delay or even prevent that bypass, wouldn't you take me up on it? I'm completely serious. The effectiveness of diet, exercise, supplements, and medicine in treating coronary heart disease has skyrocketed now that we've unlocked many of the metabolic secrets of coronary heart disease.

That's because we can now tailor a plan for your *individual* needs. If I treated all of my patients the same way, I'd only benefit about 30 percent of them—the 30 percent who'd achieve optimal benefit from that particular treatment path. That's not good enough, and fortunately, we can now do a lot better. With this added diagnostic information, we can isolate your specific metabolic issues and make sure you're receiving the best, most customized treatment for your cardiac type. We can now provide optimal treatment and achieve optimal results with *every single* person.

Only by customizing programs to meet patient-specific needs can we achieve optimal results. And the stakes are high—we're talking about saving lives! So that's why I don't put everyone on the same program and why I'm profoundly suspicious of any health program that advertises itself as a universal cure-all. We must take into account all the information an individual's personal Cardiac Fingerprint presents to us—in order to cure all.

Finally we are poised to get a true foothold against cardiac disease. When we're treating *you* and your specific set of risk factors, it's not hit or miss—

we gain a realistic chance of stabilizing, improving, possibly even beginning to *reverse* your coronary heart disease! And we can seriously reduce your risk of a cardiac event as a result.

THE LIFESTYLE PRESCRIPTIONS

As you'll notice, three essential parts of these Prescriptions are, in fact, lifestyle oriented: weight control, changes to diet, and also exercise.

Many of my newer patients, especially those who have strong family histories of coronary heart disease, ask me if lifestyle changes can really help or if they're just window dressing. As you know by now, I strongly believe that coronary heart disease, even in those who do have a powerful genetic predisposition, is nearly 100 percent preventable or treatable. There's good reason for the nutrition and exercise legs of my program to bear as much weight as medication does. I want my readers to understand, just as my patients do, that for me, these lifestyle Prescriptions are every bit as important and as effective as any medication I may prescribe.

Lifestyle changes *do* work—sometimes dramatically. But the lifestyle changes you establish need to be consistently maintained, and you'll see that their effect is cumulative. One change (a 10-pound weight loss, for instance) may cause only a minor change in LDL cholesterol; let's say five points. That five points isn't going to save your life. But if you make five more changes that each give you another five points, then that's a 30-point swing—and that *is* the kind of change that can save your life.

For a great many of you, these lifestyle changes will be the only parts of the program you will need. Many of the most popular and the most expensive drugs have exactly the same effects as lifestyle changes; in fact, in some cases, lifestyle changes can actually render lifelong drug therapy unnecessary. Statins lower LDL by up-regulating the liver's LDL receptors. So does a high-fiber, low-fat diet. Niacin stimulates the system that chews up triglyceride-rich VLDLs, lowering triglycerides and raising HDL. So can an appropriate diet and exercise program.

And obviously, the benefits of weight control, diet, and exercise on your body extend far beyond your heart—these are major factors in preventing many kinds of diseases or conditions. They're less expensive than medication, and all the side effects are positive. Let me say it again: It's crucial that you put as much stock in the Nutrition and Exercise Prescriptions as you do in the medicines that may also be part of your treatment.

This emphasis on lifestyle shouldn't be misconstrued as an argument *against* drugs—medications are some of the most effective weapons in our fight against cardiac disease, and if medication is necessary, it can be extraordinarily useful. But I always want you to augment your medical therapy with lifestyle changes. Whenever it's possible, I prefer my patients to control their metabolic issues through their lifestyles rather than through lifelong drug therapy.

INDIVIDUAL TREATMENT PRESCRIPTIONS

In the following section of the book, you will receive your individualized treatment Prescription—a "prescription" not just for medication, but for a heart-healthy life. Remember, no one can prescribe a plan for you without first examining you and taking your full history. The Prescriptions outlined in this book are guides for you and your physician to discuss prior to making any changes. Now that you have a completed Cardiac Fingerprint, it's time to use that information to build an action plan that's tailor-fit to your cardiac profile.

Before making out any prescription, your doctor evaluates you based on a wide range of factors—your weight, medical history, any history of allergies, physical reasons you may not tolerate certain types of exercise, and so on. Whatever treatment he ends up prescribing will be precise and targeted specifically to you. In my view, that same precision should also be the goal when it comes to "prescribing" diet and exercise.

The *prescription* is the key. If I simply tell patients "to diet" or "to exercise," in most cases, they're not going to get the results they need (and I want) to see. This doesn't mean that diet and exercise don't work—only that the prescription was off. The directive was too vague and too general. Prescribing the same diet and exercise plan for everyone isn't much better. A treatment plan must be targeted toward the specific combination of conditions you want to treat or it just won't accomplish what you want it to. Sure, a generalized plan is going to be right for some people by default, but it's going to be wrong for a whole lot of others. And in the same way that the wrong drug won't make you better, the wrong diet, exercise, or supplementation plan won't help you to adequately prevent or treat coronary heart disease either. That's just common sense.

I've said that diet and exercise can have as powerful a therapeutic impact on your heart health as conventional medical treatment paths—and that's true, as long as they're the right plans. These Advanced Metabolic Markers give us the blueprint for the lifestyle programs that will work—everything we need to construct plans that address your particular risk profile. Now that you have the information in your complete Cardiac Fingerprint, we can get away from those generalized, standardized (and often ineffective) recommendations. We now have the information we need to "prescribe" the most effective diet, exercise, and supplement plan for you.

As you learned in chapter 4, each of these markers helps us to predict your coronary heart disease risk, and each one of these metabolic or genetic abnormalities signals a distinct problem. We also know that the majority of these problems are treatable. So the key is to isolate which markers are affected by which therapies and then come up with a plan to treat them. That's easily done. But we also know that the way these markers work together with one another can also increase your risk. Since you probably have some combination of these markers, we have to take *all* of them into account when devising that plan, in the same way that your doctor considers all of your conditions when she's prescribing a medication. Since we can now identify the enemy that is gunning for you, and predict its line of attack, we can finally contain it. Our job is to strike back, preferably before these cumulative effects have taken their toll.

That is the goal of this book, and the reason for offering a set of individualized Prescription plans tailored to your Cardiac Fingerprint.

Let's get to it: It's time to get you fitted for the Prescription plans that can help you stay heart-healthy for the rest of your life. There are four parts to the program: the Nutrition Prescription (chapter 7), the Exercise Prescription (chapter 8), the Medication Prescription (chapter 9), and the Supplement Prescription (chapter 10).

First, a word about the mechanics of getting you fitted

Your Advanced Metabolic Marker Profile is what we use to match you up with your individualized Prescription plans. That's because the plans to which you'll be assigned have been calibrated according to your personal Advanced Metabolic Marker Profile.

But don't worry. Even if you have chosen not to take the advanced marker tests, the Prescription Key will direct you to Diet and Exercise Plans that will get you started on the road to heart health.

In each of the Prescription programs (Nutrition, Exercise, Medication, Supplements), you'll find three different plans. Each plan is calibrated to address specific sets of metabolic issues. The way you know which of the three plans is the right one for you is to consult the Prescription Key that appears at the start of each program. This Key will assign you to the plan that is appropriate for you and your specific combination of metabolic concerns. It's easy: All you have to do is refer back to your Quick Reference Chart (see page 91) and then plug your results into the Key to find out where you fit.

Next to each Prescription Key, you'll always find four Advanced Metabolic Markers, because in each instance we are isolating the four specific Advanced Metabolic Markers that are most impacted by the program at hand. There are Diet Markers, Exercise Markers, Medication Markers, and Supplement Markers.

When I say these Advanced Metabolic Markers are impacted by the programs here's what I mean. Take as an example someone whose lab results reveal that they have a dangerous LDL pattern B profile. Often an individual can convert to the less dangerous LDL pattern A simply by making dietary changes! This particular metabolic imbalance is very strongly affected by nutrition, so the Diet Plan you follow can have tremendous therapeutic impact on this serious condition.

Bear in mind, however, that the therapeutic impact of food can work both ways. Just as people can convert from the dangerous LDL pattern B into the more healthy LDL pattern A simply by eating the right diet, it is just as possible for some people to begin to convert from a healthy LDL pattern A into the more unhealthy LDL pattern B on the wrong diet—even a low-fat diet that appears to be perfectly healthy! This is why it is so important to get tested and, once tested, to get yourself on the right plans for you.

Just as the right Diet Plan can affect certain metabolic imbalances, so can exercise, medication, and supplements. Depending on your Advanced Metabolic Marker Profile, the way you eat, how you exercise, and what medications and supplements you are taking can all work to help (or worsen!) your underlying metabolic condition. But we have to match the right Advanced Metabolic Markers with the right treatment. Different sets of markers therefore control each of the four programs within the book. In this way, we can truly customize each Prescription for maximum impact and direct you to the ones that will be most appropriate for you.

Before proceeding with the Prescriptions, I'd like to emphasize again that you should always begin a new therapy only under the supervision of a physician who is fully up to date on both your family medical history and your own medical history. Even something as seemingly benign as a diet and exercise program can be dangerous if it's not supervised by a medical professional. These programs are not meant to serve as substitutes for proper medical care. They are intended as recommendations, to give you and your doctor a launchpad for a discussion about more personalized therapy.

That said, you and your doctor are about to take a very important first step in your own personal fight against coronary heart disease! Let's move on now to the specific Prescriptions, beginning with Nutrition.

7

THE NUTRITION PRESCRIPTION

AN INTRODUCTION TO DIET AND YOUR HEART

DIET IS THE BRIDESMAID of cardiac health. You don't need a medical degree to know that there's a correlation between that nightly ice cream habit and those steadily worsening angiograms! But while plenty of lip service gets paid to changing our eating habits and shedding those extra pounds, diet always seems to take a backseat to medical intervention when we want to see rapid results.

Diet shouldn't be the last thing we seriously address when we want to get better—it should be the *first*.

Part of the problem has been that the standard dietary recommendations generally prescribed to cardiac patients don't work for everyone—a problem that, as you'll see, we now have the tools to improve. Past failures were often the result of the wrong diet for that specific individual, plain and simple. That failure must not, however, be taken as reason to abandon diet as a viable tool in the battle against cardiac disease. The standard dietary recommendations didn't work because they were overly standardized, and an off-the-rack diet only fits *some* of us well! The same goes for a cookie-cutter approach to weight loss. Putting everyone on the same dietary protocol often results in failure and frustration.

So it's no wonder that with all the effective medications we have at our fingertips, doctors and patients are opting for pills over dietary changes to treat the symptoms of coronary heart disease. But we can't forget that diet itself is one of the most powerful tools in our battle against coronary heart disease and its underlying causes—not to mention one with far fewer associated complications compared to drug therapy.

In fact, today we can do some truly amazing things with diet! With our newfound ability to isolate and target your particular constellation of cardiac issues, nutrition can be a major weapon against coronary heart disease. When I put my patients on individualized diet and nutrition programs that have been targeted to attack their particular metabolic marker abnormalities, the results can be tremendous. That's why I'm dragging diet out onto the dance floor by making it the very first Prescription that we address.

BOB'S STORY

Bob is a 64-year-old man. Last year, he thought he was in relatively good health but was carrying about 30 extra pounds when he was diagnosed with high blood pressure. His doctor immediately put him on a beta-blocker, one of the oldest and most effective medications we use to control hypertension.

Bob mentioned the diagnosis and new medication to his daughter, who knew something about hypertension, and in time-honored, bossy-daughter fashion, she started to take control. You see, at no point during this first appointment, or in any of the ones that followed, did this doctor mention nutrition or weight loss as contributing factors to Bob's high blood pressure. Fortunately, his daughter knew better.

Now Bob wasn't eating at fast food restaurants every day; in fact, his diet was relatively moderate. But, like many of my patients, he simply needed a better understanding of how the food he ate was affecting his health. He had never really paid much attention to calories, or what distinguished different kinds of fats. He didn't know that there might be a correlation between a high-sodium diet and high blood pressure, and he had no idea how much sodium was in his diet anyway. He didn't overuse the salt shaker and had no clue that some of his favorite foods, like peanut butter, were loaded with sodium—not to mention calories and, in some brands, unhealthy saturated and trans fats.

So Bob and his daughter started at the very beginning. The first stop was the grocery store, where she taught him to read food labels. She also taught him to rethink portion size and to count calories in a very general way. He learned about whole grains and the different kinds of fat, and they found a local store that sold sodium-free canned tomatoes so he wouldn't have to stop making his beloved marinara sauce. He started a regular exercise program for the first time since his thirties, watched what (and how much) he ate, and lost those 30 pounds.

Luckily, he happened to be one of the people whose blood pressure responds well to weight loss and a low-sodium diet. Today, his blood pressure is down, well within normal range, and at his next appointment, he's going to ask his doctor to consider backing him off the beta-blocker.

What went wrong?

I tell this story for a number of reasons. I'm sad that Bob's doctor didn't make the issue of diet and weight loss a number-one priority for this patient right off the bat. But I'm not surprised. Our healthcare system isn't set up to encourage physicians to take a holistic approach toward our patients' health. As doctors, we're discouraged from spending time with our patients and driven to find the most cost-effective solution to their health problems, which often means cramming as many people as possible into a single clinic day. People often have to switch physicians every time their health insurance changes, so there's often little continuity in the relationship between doctor and patient.

Now not every patient will respond to a low-sodium diet as well as Bob did. So a doctor responsible for a hypertensive patient's care must monitor progress carefully to determine whether a nutritional strategy is really working. In other words, going for a less aggressive treatment approach will require more aggressive follow-up, and that added commitment is often seen as a less attractive option, by both patient and doctor, than the quicker fix of prescribing a pill. Medication is popular because it can be accomplished with minimal time spent educating and supervising the patient, it is frequently effective in lowering blood pressure, and often has a high rate of patient compliance. Still, quickest is not always best. Just look at Bob.

Without his daughter's intervention, Bob might have spent the rest of his life dependent on medication to treat a condition that he was perfectly capable of controlling himself. Instead, he took steps that not only successfully addressed his condition, but that have positive ramifications for his whole heart—and his overall health.

It's true: Dietary changes are major lifestyle changes. They do require some education and motivation on your part. Someone has to take you to a grocery store and teach you how to read a label—or you have to do that work yourself—and then you have to integrate that information into your everyday life. From a physician's standpoint, I also know very well how frustrating it is when you tell someone to lose weight, or just to change his diet, and he doesn't.

But I have more faith in my patients—and in my readers—than Bob's doctor did. I know that if I explain to you why certain dietary choices are endangering your health and then give you the tools to make healthier choices, most of you will give it a try. And that's all I need, because once you get the ball rolling, you are going to look and feel terrific—and you're going to get a big kick out of the look on your doctor's face when he sees your new cholesterol and Advanced Metabolic Marker numbers improving! This is what I mean by you taking control.

Losing 20 pounds, or cutting sugar or sodium, is never going to be as quick and easy as taking a pill. But the other, and most important, reason to share Bob's story is simply to demonstrate how great the results can be. Bob has essentially cured himself of one of the most significant risk factors for a cardiac event. The beta-blocker was effective for moving him out of the immediate danger zone, but now he's going to be able to replicate that drug's results—without the drug!—for the rest of his life. Even if Bob hadn't been totally successful through diet alone, his efforts almost certainly would have reduced the dose of medication he needed.

And if you ask him, you'll find that Bob isn't complaining. He's not pushing lettuce around a plate and whining about it; in fact, he didn't have to give up anything he couldn't live without. He looks better. He feels better physically and emotionally because he's more in control of his health. He's going to save a lot of money when he goes off the beta-blocker (either for himself or for his insurance company), and he'll have the peace of mind of knowing that he's not dependent on medication.

THE NUTRITION PRESCRIPTION

All the tools you'll need to achieve your own great results are contained here in the Nutrition Prescription. There are three steps to the process.

First, I'll walk you through some nutrition basics in the section that follows. There, I'll review the basic nutrition "building blocks" that will help you learn how to eat your way to a healthier heart. After that, we turn to a section dedicated expressly to those of you who are carrying a few extra pounds (and who isn't?). I'll show you how to determine if you're overweight, explain what those extra pounds mean for your heart, and give you practical tips and easily adopted advice on how to get rid of them. Although this section is targeted to those readers who need to lose weight, there's a lot of general information on healthy eating, and I'd encourage everyone to read it.

Once you've got those two sections under your belt, you'll be ready for the third and final step of the Nutrition Prescription: finding and following the customized Diet Plan that's tailored for you and your heart. Here's where we take the information from your own personal Cardiac Fingerprint and use it to determine precisely which diet is best for your personal cardiac makeup.

So let's get started!

NUTRITION BASICS

With the amount of time, energy, and money thrown at diet in America, you'd think we'd all look like Olympic athletes, each of us sporting a set of dazzlingly clean and shiny arterial passages. Instead—well, we look like we look. With so much information at our disposal, how can we be anything but the leanest, meanest versions of ourselves?

The question may contain the answer. The volume of the information we're bombarded with on television, in books and magazines, and anecdotally is completely overwhelming! Just sorting through the contradictory claims put forth by experts—many of them medical doctors—can be a full-time job.

Sure, we all know somebody who's gloating about losing 40 pounds on a diet of nothing but steak, eggs, cheese, and bacon—but it's hard to ignore the little voice in the back of our heads that is wondering just how healthy such a diet can possibly be over the long term. Other people do seem to be controlling their weight successfully, but it's a miracle they eat at all, considering how unappetizing and bland the minuscule portion of food in front of them looks. At the same time, many of you have tried to improve your own cholesterol numbers through diet, only to find that you're going hungry—and despite all the sacrifice, there's been little or no improvement in your blood test results after all.

So what's the solution? In this area, as in so many others, we're running up against the same one-size-fits-all problem. We're all physiologically different, and the way we respond to treatment is different. Diet is no exception. But how can we sort through the mountains of information out there to get to the Diet Plan that's going to work best for us? And how can we make sure that the plan we choose is the *healthiest* one for each of us—not just a quick-fix way to shed pounds, one that will strain our hearts while we're losing weight, and soon find us gaining it all back anyway?

In the Nutrition Prescription in this book, I've applied the newest science to the only question that really matters: What's the healthiest way for *you* to eat? My goal is to customize dietary programs for you and your personal cardiac profile. The right fit makes all the difference.

And my aim is not simply to put you on a diet, per se. When you finish reading this book, you will have a complete tool kit, one that enables you to make changes in your lifestyle that will positively impact your health throughout your life. I've included, for example, 1 week of sample meal plans in the Nutrition Prescription, with the understanding that that 1 week will be just the beginning. It's an old story: If you give a man a fish, you give him dinner; if you teach a man to fish, you give him dinner for the rest of his life (and a heart-healthy one, at that!). I want you to understand the nutritional principles that make sense for your particular Diet Plan, so that you'll have the power to create endless variations of your own delicious and heart-healthy meals long after that week is up. This crash course in nutrition is all you'll need.

THE BASIC BUILDING BLOCKS

Contrary to the impression you might get from the popular media, nutrition isn't tremendously complicated; there's no voodoo magic to the way it works. The foods we eat are made up of building blocks—fats, carbohydrates, and protein—and those building blocks have fairly predictable effects on our bodies. But some of us inherit sensitivities or resistances to certain of these building blocks, and that explains why different people on the same diets can have such wildly different results, even though the building blocks themselves remain constant.

We'll talk more about these sensitivities and resistances when we look at your own Cardiac Fingerprint. Let's focus right now on those basic building blocks and how they affect your body.

Fats

Fats have long been cast as the number-one artery-clogging, obesity-causing villains of American health. As a result, our supermarket shelves are bursting with low-fat and fat-free products.

The truth about fats, of course, is a little more complicated. Fat isn't the enemy it's been made out to be. First of all, your body needs fat. Fat is the material in the cells that stores and provides energy; it protects us from the cold, acts as a shock absorber for our organs, and keeps skin healthy. So our diets must have some fat in them.

Let's take a closer look. What is a blood fat, the kind that's measured by the common blood test? It's a triglyceride: a particle with three (this is where the *tri-* comes from) fatty acids attached to it. It looks like Poseidon's trident. These fatty acids can be saturated and unsaturated, and that's one way we differentiate between fats. As you'll see, the difference between the effects of saturated and unsaturated fats on your arteries is dramatic. Fat isn't the enemy, but the *wrong kind* of fat can be.

Unsaturated Fats

In general, unsaturated fats are considerably better for you than saturated fats. Most vegetable oils (with the exception of the tropical oils, such as coconut and palm-kernel oil) are unsaturated. A good way to tell the difference fast? Unsaturated fats are liquid at room temperature.

Within the general category of unsaturated fats, there are actually two different types: monounsaturated and polyunsaturated.

Monounsaturated fats. Studies have been done on diets that replace saturated fats with monounsaturated fats, and they show a substantial reduction in the "bad" LDL cholesterol. You may have read or heard about the Mediter-

MONOUNSATURATED FATS

Major sources. Olive and canola oils; walnuts and almonds.

Healthy choices. These monounsaturated fats are the healthy-choice fats that you should be using at home for cooking and adding to foods (like salad dressings). All fats, even the "good ones," carry a lot of calories compared to the other building blocks—about 100 calories per tablespoon. Be mindful of this, especially if your weight is an issue.

OMEGA-6 FATTY ACIDS

Major sources. Safflower, sunflower, corn, and soybean oils. The generic "vegetable oil" at the supermarket is probably one or a combination of these types of oils. Avoid buying these oils for cooking or adding to food.

Healthy choices. Since you're already getting a lot of these oils in prepared foods, we suggest that you don't cook with them at home. Choose a monounsaturated fat like canola or olive oil instead.

ranean diet, which relies heavily on olive oil, nuts, and other "fatty" foods. These fats are mostly monounsaturated, which appears to account for the much lower coronary heart disease rates in countries that follow these diets.

Polyunsaturated fats. The other kind of unsaturated fats is polyunsaturated fats. And there are actually two important kinds of polyunsaturated fats: the omega-6s and the omega-3s.

The **omega-6 fatty acids** are found in vegetable oils such as corn, soybean, and safflower oils. The food industry uses a lot of soybean oil, so you're probably already getting a lot of these omega-6s in your diet. The good news is that they do lower blood cholesterol a little. The bad news is that they have a lowering effect not only on the "bad" LDL cholesterol, but also on the "good" HDL cholesterol. For this reason and others (diets extremely high in these fats have also been linked to a high oxidation potential), we suggest that you go lightly in your consumption of them. An easy way to do this is to make sure that they're not among the fats you use at home for cooking and adding to food.

Omega-3 fatty acids are also polyunsaturated fatty acids, but they appear to have much more powerful cardiac benefits than their omega-6 cousins. And of the omega-3s, the most beneficial of those are eicosapentaenoic acid (EPA) and docosahexaenoic acid (DHA).

These omega-3s are nutrients that the body can't make on its own, so we need to get them from food. The best food source for these particular omega-3s is fish oils. (We'll discuss them in much greater detail in chapter 10 when I

OMEGA-3 FATTY ACIDS

Major sources. Fish, especially fatty ones, like salmon, herring, sardines, and lake trout. Vegetable sources include canola, walnut, and flaxseed oils, wheat germ, and soybeans, although the fatty acids found in them may not share the same benefits as the omega-3s found in fish.

Healthy choices. I recommend that you make fish a regular feature of your diet. Try for two fish meals a week, but add more if you'd like. Avoid fried fish in restaurants and fast food places: It's usually low in omega-3s, and the fats these fish are fried in make them high in unhealthy trans fats. You can also sprinkle flaxseed on your cereal and include it in baked goods. Use canola oil for cooking, baking, and salad dressings.

talk about supplements.) The omega-3s in fish and fish oils have been linked to reduced rates of coronary heart disease. Studies show that they reduce triglycerides, raise HDL, and have a host of other heart-friendly side effects. They reduce the risk of blood clots and relax the arteries so they're less likely to clamp down unexpectedly, and they appear to help regulate the electrical signals the heart muscle sends, decreasing the likelihood of irregular heart rhythms.

It can sometimes be pretty difficult to get the amount of fish oils you need from eating fish, and we'll discuss some of your other options in chapter 10. But I would encourage everyone to add more fish to their diets. It's a terrific, lower-calorie substitute for red meat, and the fat you'll find in fish is much better for you than the saturated fats you'll find in red meat. In fact, I've often wondered how much of the benefits of a diet rich in fish can be boiled down to this simple truth: A diet rich in fish is a diet that's not rich in hamburger.

Saturated Fats

Saturated fats are the "bad" fats. They'll raise your LDL cholesterol level more than anything else, including the cholesterol you get from food. How can you tell them apart from their heart-healthy unsaturated cousins? A good rule of thumb: Saturated fats are solid at room temperature. That white chunk the butcher cuts off a piece of steak? Lard? Butter? These are all saturated fats, and consuming them has a powerful and adverse effect on your blood cholesterol levels and heart health.

As you may have noticed, the three examples above all come from animals, and most saturated fats do. There are a few notable exceptions: cocoa butter and palm, palm-kernel, and coconut oils. Vegetable or no, these are just as bad for you as lard and butter!

A number of studies in different populations have shown the link between diets high in saturated fat and coronary heart disease. The countries (and the United States is right up there) with the highest intakes of saturated fats are the countries with the highest rates of coronary heart disease. In fact, one of these studies looked at the diets of Japanese men living in three different locations: Japan, Hawaii, and the United States. The farther east the men moved, the more saturated fat they ate, and the more saturated fat they ate, the higher their cholesterol and the higher their rates of coronary heart disease.

You don't have to cut saturated fats out of your diet completely, but we do suggest that you limit the foods that contain them.

SATURATED FATS

Major sources. Beef, pork, lamb, and chicken; whole-milk cheese, ice cream, whole milk, and butter; cocoa butter and palm, palm-kernel, and coconut oils.

Healthy choices. Trim all visible fat off your meat. Choose lean cuts (tenderloin, sirloin, round). When eating poultry, choose white (breast) meat more often than dark (leg, thigh), and don't eat the skin. Choose low-fat or fat-free versions of your favorite dairy foods: nonfat or low-fat milk and cheese, ice milk or frozen yogurt instead of ice cream. (But be cautious about the sugar content!) Choose a canola-based tub margarine instead of butter. Avoid products containing tropical oils.

Trans Fats

Food companies love to use saturated fats in products because they give food a much longer shelf life than unsaturated fats do. But when John Q. Public started reading labels and rejecting products containing these saturated tropical oils, the food companies had to come up with something else, and that something else was a process called **hydrogenation.**

Hydrogenation is a chemical process that turns less-harmful unsaturated fats into fats that behave much like saturated fats. Good for the shelf life of a product, not so good for your arteries. These hydrogenated fats contain **trans fats,** or trans saturated fatty acids. You've probably heard about them—they've (deservedly) received quite a bit of bad press over the last couple of years. Not only do they raise your LDL, but they've also been shown to lower HDL, and trans fats may also increase your Lp(a). In a study of approximately 90,000 women, the women who ate the most trans fats had a 27 percent higher risk of coronary heart disease than the ones who ate the least.

The big problem with trans fats is that they aren't listed on food labels. So you have no idea if the food you're choosing has them, unless you read the ingredient list, looking for hydrogenated or partially hydrogenated oils. These are dangerous because they're sneaky; you're in the grocery store comparing product labels—let's say crackers—and you know that saturated fats gener-

TRANS FATS

Major sources. Vegetable shortenings; margarines, especially stick margarines; hydrogenated peanut butter (any kind that doesn't separate when left to stand); commercially prepared baked goods such as pies, cakes, cookies, crackers, pastries, doughnuts, and potato chips; fast foods.

■ *Avoid the foods listed above as much as possible.*

Healthy choices. Choose a trans fat–free margarine (these will be clearly marked; there are a few currently on the market) or a tub margarine, which will have fewer trans fats.

ally come from animals, so you go with the product that contains vegetable oils. Gotcha! If those vegetable oils are actually hydrogenated fats, they're just as bad or worse for your heart than their animal-derived alternatives. See the box on the opposite page for a partial list of foods that contain them; avoid these as much as possible.

How much fat should I be eating?

The American Heart Association currently recommends that people keep fat below 30 percent of their total daily calories.

While anything that encourages Americans to eat less saturated fat is a good thing, we know that we can do better than this kind of one-size-fits-all recommendation. Like everything else, diet recommendations should be individualized depending on your genetic makeup and underlying metabolic sensitivities. In reality, 30 percent of total calories is too high for some people, too low for others.

Yes, you heard right: too low in fat! In a study on 105 men following high-fat and low-fat diets, 36 men changed from a relatively harmless LDL pattern A to a dangerously atherogenic LDL pattern B on the low-fat diet. Even the men who remained pattern A throughout the study also experienced a shift in LDL particle size from large LDL particles to the more hazardous small, dense particles—not quite enough to turn them into pattern Bs, but certainly heading in that direction. So too little fat can be as big a problem for certain people as too much can be for others.

In the Nutrition Prescription, we'll interpret your personal Cardiac Fingerprint in order to arrive at the best dietary recommendations for your heart, complete with specific breakdowns by percentage of the amounts of the various building blocks you need to achieve maximum health.

Carbohydrates

Carbohydrates have been at the center of the recent "diet wars." Are these basic building blocks making us obese, or are they actually the only way out of the mess we're in?

Like everything else, the answer is both simpler and more complex than it's been portrayed. Here are the basics: Carbohydrates are the body's rapid source of energy. All carbohydrates are composed of sugar units. Chemically, carbs can be classified as either simple or complex. Simple carbohydrates are commonly referred to as sugars. Practically speaking, think of this as fruit juices, dried fruit, soda, muffins, pies, etc. Complex carbohydrates, so called because their structure is much longer than the sugars, are the starches and most of the fibers. Examples include whole grain products, pasta, and potatoes.

We can digest simple carbs more quickly than complex carbs. Sugars get absorbed into our bloodstream very rapidly and can cause a dramatic spike—and then sometimes a dramatic fall—in blood-sugar level. Since most of the complex carbohydrates usually get broken down more slowly, they're absorbed into the bloodstream more slowly, and they provide a more level supply of energy.

Sugars can also increase our blood triglyceride levels. Complex carbohydrates generally don't increase triglyceride levels as much, but if you're on a very-high-carbohydrate diet, even though you are eating complex carbohydrates, you may see an increase because of the sheer volume of the carbs you're consuming.

The Glycemic Index

So "simple" and "complex" gives us the first level of categorization we use to think and talk about carbs. We're now able to get even more specific. About 20 years ago, researchers started measuring the way different foods affected blood sugar—how long foods took to be absorbed, how high they drove blood-sugar levels, and for how long. The result of this research was the glycemic index. Foods with a high glycemic index act like glucose (a sugar—and sugars do rate very high on the index). These high-glycemic foods raise blood-sugar levels higher and for a longer time than an equal amount of a low-glycemic food. High-glycemic foods are absorbed quickly, followed by a surge in blood sugar. This leads to a hormonal overcorrection, which dumps a ton of insulin into your bloodstream and may bring your blood sugar too low. That's why you feel an energy boost immediately after a sweet treat—and feel ready for a nap about an hour later.

Low-glycemic-index foods are mainly unrefined, complex carbohydrates, and they're absorbed into the bloodstream more slowly. When we strip a grain of its fibrous husk and nutritious germ—as we do to make white rice from brown, for instance—we turn it from a low-glycemic-index food into a high-glycemic-index food. Brown rice has a low glycemic index; instant white rice is really high.

Most refined, high-carbohydrate foods—like white bread—have a high glycemic index. However, starchy vegetables, such as potatoes, are also high on the scale. Most whole grains, vegetables, fruits, and legumes have low glycemic indexes. In order to have the slowest, most even release of energy into your bloodstream, choose low-glycemic-index foods whenever possible.

In other words, all carbohydrates are not created equal. The point is not to cut carbs completely, but to make healthier choices about the ones you do

CARBOHYDRATES

Major sources. Rice, oats, wheat, barley, quinoa; bread, pita, crackers, cake, cookies; all vegetables and legumes (potatoes, peas, corn); sugars

Healthy choices. Eat sparingly from the simple carbohydrate category and much more generously from the complex carbohydrate category. From that list, make an effort to choose foods low on the glycemic index, such as legumes, milk, barley, and most fruits and vegetables. Remember to have at least five servings of vegetables a day, and add legumes to meals whenever possible. Also, choose whole grains over white ones; multigrain bread over white; brown rice over white. Choose whole grain, unsweet-ened cereal over sugar cereal. Avoid excess sugar and products containing sugar. If it tastes sweet, it almost certainly contains a simple sugar.

eat. Almost every refined carbohydrate has an unrefined alternative. And you don't even have to give up those refined carbohydrates entirely—you just have to put them in the "rare" category.

Carbohydrates and Coronary Heart Disease

So what's the correlation between coronary heart disease and carbohydrates? Populations that eat a lot of unrefined carbs also tend to be populations with low risk of coronary heart disease. Of course, high-carbohydrate diets also tend to be low-fat diets, so it's difficult to separate those two variables.

Another thing is clear, though—the carbohydrates that people are eating in countries with low risk of coronary heart disease are unrefined and have a low glycemic index. These people aren't dodging coronary heart disease by pigging out exclusively on sugary doughnuts and white bread. They're eating more unrefined grains and vegetables than meat—or doughnuts.

Numerous studies have shown that increases in carbs can lead to elevated triglycerides and decreases in HDL. Again, this has much to do with the kind of carbohydrates people are eating. The simple carbohydrates, like sucrose (table sugar) and fructose (fruit sugar), have been linked to an increased production of triglycerides.

So we know that you should focus on complex carbohydrates. But how much is too much? How much carbohydrate you should consume, like how much fat, depends on your particular genetic proclivities and underlying metabolic conditions, so we'll be able to make individualized recommendations in the Nutrition Prescription section.

Some very-low-fat diets, like those advocated by some physicians, contain such high amounts of dietary carbohydrates (75 to 80 percent of calories) that they may also lead to an increase in triglycerides in some individuals— just because of the volume of carbohydrates they have to consume. For certain people, that can be very dangerous. High-carbohydrate, low-fat diets have also been shown to encourage people to convert to the dangerous small LDL pattern B profile. So we need to look closely at your profile and customize your carbohydrate recommendation to make sure you're doing the best thing for your heart.

Protein

Proteins are the last building block of the three.

What is a protein? It's a chain of amino acids, like a railroad train made up of amino acid "cars" that can twist into a variety of complex shapes. The body contains 20 different kinds of amino acids, and these can be connected in a multitude of different combinations to form thousands of different types of proteins. These proteins really are the building blocks of the body's structures, such as your skin, organs, tendons, and muscles. In fact, within each cell, proteins are constantly being made—without them, your body can't grow or heal.

How much protein should I be eating?

The quantity of the protein you eat doesn't seem to have much effect on your cholesterol level, but the *source* of the protein you eat does. Meat, eggs, and dairy products are very good sources of protein—but they can also be very good sources of unhealthy saturated fats, which will increase your blood cholesterol, so don't forget to incorporate information about fat into your protein choices. Leaner cuts of meat and white-meat poultry are high in protein but

PROTEIN

Major sources. Meat, fish, poultry; dairy products; legumes, beans, and peas; soy.

Healthy choices. Choose proteins that are comparatively low in saturated fat: fish, white-meat skinless poultry, lean cuts of meat, egg whites, low-fat dairy products, and low-fat soy products. Whenever possible, replace meat with soy and high-protein vegetables, like beans.

relatively low in saturated fat. Soy and beans are very good vegetable-derived protein sources; they're not only lower in fat than their meat counterparts, but contain better kinds of fat as well as other essential vitamins and health-promoting antioxidants. Moreover, soy has a whole host of scientifically proven, heart-healthy benefits. The U.S. Food and Drug Administration recently recommended that Americans consume 25 grams of soy protein a day. That's four servings! I know that sounds like a lot, but if you substitute soy protein for animal protein whenever possible, you'll be doing your heart a world of good.

CHOLESTEROL

Where does cholesterol fit into all of this? Cholesterol isn't technically a building block, but since it's so central to all conversations about coronary heart disease, I'm going to address it in this section. Cholesterol has been cast as the villain in the coronary heart disease story, but did you know that you need cholesterol to do a lot of good things too? For example, cholesterol is a basic building block for very important hormones such as estrogen and testosterone, and it's an important component of cell structure. The problem starts when you have an abundance of LDL cholesterol or, worse yet, an abundance of small LDL cholesterol, which can promote arterial blockage in ways we have discussed.

As we know, you get cholesterol from two different sources: Your body manufactures it and you eat it in food. You make all the cholesterol your body

CHOLESTEROL

Major sources. Eggs; meats, fish, and poultry; organ meats such as brains, kidney, sweetbreads, liver; shrimp and squid; whole milk, cheese, and ice cream.

Healthy choices. Choose egg-white products. Choose oysters, clams, or lobster over shrimp and squid. Choose fat-free or low-fat versions of dairy products.

needs, so let's take a closer look at the cholesterol you eat, which we call **dietary cholesterol.**

Dietary cholesterol is found exclusively in animal products: eggs, meat, fish, poultry, and dairy products. Eggs and organ meats (liver, sweetbreads, brains, and kidneys) are the most concentrated sources of cholesterol. Although cholesterol is different from saturated fat, it's often found in foods that also contain saturated fat. This is a good rule of thumb, but it's not infallible; high concentrations of cholesterol can also be found in foods that are low in fat. Liver, for example, is very high in cholesterol, although it's low in fat.

There are also products in food that look like cholesterol but have no effect on your lipid levels. For a long time, we warned people away from shellfish like oysters, clams, lobster, scallops, and crab because they were high in these cholesterol look-alikes. Now we know that they're actually all lower in cholesterol than we had previously thought and contain very little fat. (Not all shellfish got the stamp of approval, though: Shrimp, prawns, and squid are still very high in cholesterol.)

How much cholesterol can I eat?

It has long been believed that eating cholesterol raises your blood cholesterol. In fact, the studies on this subject are mixed. We do believe that dietary cholesterol raises cholesterol levels, but we now believe that individuals react differently to dietary cholesterol, based both on the kinds of fat they eat with the cholesterol and their inherited responsiveness.

That said, you'd do well to avoid high amounts of dietary cholesterol. When you eat too much cholesterol, your body turns off those LDL receptors on the liver, the ones that are taking all that LDL cholesterol out of the bloodstream. The fewer active LDL receptors you have, the more LDL cholesterol you'll have left in your bloodstream—and the higher your numbers and your risk of coronary heart disease will be. Studies have also shown that large amounts of dietary cholesterol increase the number of apo Bs you make, which means that whether you have large or small LDL, you have more of them.

ALCOHOL: WILL A GLASS A DAY KEEP THE DOCTOR AWAY?

You might already be familiar with the French Paradox: As anyone who has traveled to Paris knows, the French certainly aren't afraid of saturated fat and cholesterol. They eat butter, pâté, red meat, organ meats, butter-rich pastries, creamy sauces—and yet they have a significantly lower rate of coronary artery disease than Americans do.

Some researchers believe that this is linked to a higher overall consumption of alcohol in France; several studies have shown that people who drink moderate amounts of alcohol (two units of beer, wine, or liquor a day) have higher "good" HDL cholesterol and reductions in death from coronary artery disease. Furthermore, the French drink a great deal of red wine, which contains both tannins and polyphenols, chemicals that may inhibit platelet stickiness and LDL oxidation.

A closer look at these studies is eye-opening, though. First of all, the French may not be dying from coronary heart disease, but the alcohol does take its toll: Liver disease is common, and the leading causes of death in France are automobile accidents and suicide, many of which can be linked to alcohol consumption. It also appears that the HDL cholesterol that is most increased by alcohol isn't HDL2b, the form of HDL cholesterol that has been linked to reduced coronary artery disease. So while the increase in HDL looks nice on paper, it may not actually be contributing in a positive way to cardiac protection.

About 10 percent of the world population has an inherited difference in the gene for an enzyme called alcohol dehydrogenase, which metabolizes alcohol in your body. These lucky people have a greater increase in HDL than most people and have a correspondingly lower risk of coronary heart disease. Don't get too happy: The odds are that you're not one of these people.

Alcohol has a negative impact on the heart in other ways as well. It can dra-

FIBER

Fiber's also not a building block, but it's a major player in the nutritional fight against coronary heart disease. Just about everyone can afford to eat more fiber, particularly people who are concerned about their hearts. There's very basic evidence for this: There's less coronary heart disease in the population in countries with high-fiber diets.

matically increase triglycerides, which increases cardiovascular risk, and more than two drinks a day have been linked to increases in blood pressure.

There was a very compelling study done in the United States that showed that people who drank more alcohol had less coronary heart disease, and people everywhere raised their glasses to the results. I believe (and there's scientific evidence to support this) that there's another, chicken-or-egg explanation for the results they saw, though: Alcohol may have had nothing to do with it. Everyone knows that the last thing you feel like doing when you get sick is drinking, especially with a serious illness. The people who were getting sick, got sick—and as they got sick, they stopped drinking. So it wasn't that the alcohol was protecting them, just that it was the first thing to go when they started getting ill.

And what about that French Paradox? Well, it might be the wine, but there are too many other variables to draw real conclusions. First of all, the French eat more fruits and vegetables than we do, and the ones they eat are fresher, which increases their vitamin content. They eat more seafood than we do. The animals they eat tend to be leaner, so they contain less fat. The French also eat a wider variety of foods than Americans, which means that they get more nutrients and limit the toxins they get from one food or another. And the French portion size is considerably smaller than the American one.

I'm not advocating temperance, but it's not yet clear to me that there's a strong argument for drinking alcohol to improve your cardiovascular health. Obviously, if you have a problem with alcohol, you should seek help to stop drinking immediately. If you don't drink, don't start. If you have serious heart problems, diabetes, or high triglycerides, you shouldn't drink at all. Everyone else should do it in moderation, if they so choose—which means no more than two drinks a day for men and one a day for women.

Fiber can't be broken down by the body, so it passes through the digestive system basically unchanged. Americans eat a very compact, calorie-rich, low-fiber diet—you'd have to eat a lot of vegetables to match the number of calories you get from a hamburger patty the size of your fist, and you'd get a lot more fiber from the vegetables. In countries where the diet is lower in fat and higher in fiber, rates of coronary heart disease are lower. One of the ex-

planations for this is that soluble fiber may block the reabsorption of cholesterol in the intestines.

In another study I conducted while at Stanford University, we gave research subjects large amounts of fiber supplements, and we did see a small reduction (about 8 percent) in LDL cholesterol. Unfortunately, when you take
large amounts of fiber supplements, you may also experience uncomfortable
side effects: loose stool, diarrhea, and bowel gas. If you increase your fiber
gradually, the gas is less of a problem.

There's still a benefit from reasonably increasing your fiber intake—especially if it's combined with other cholesterol-lowering dietary strategies. The
recommendation for dietary fiber is 20 to 35 grams a day.

There are two different kinds of fiber: soluble and insoluble. The insoluble kind doesn't seem to have much of an effect on lipid levels, but even small
increases in soluble fiber can have some effect. I recommend that people increase their total fiber intake in a combination of ways. A diet that's high in
fiber is the best thing, and since the American diet does tend to be so dependent on highly processed, high-fat, calorie-rich food, it's not difficult to make
a big difference through some minor modifications.

All you have to do is to increase the number of whole grains, legumes,
fruits, and vegetables in your diet. Choose whole wheat breads and pasta instead of their refined white alternatives, make sure to eat at least five servings
of vegetables a day, add legumes to your soups and salads and a high-fiber cereal to your morning routine—for starters. Oatmeal is a great source of soluble

DIETARY FIBER

Major sources. Whole grains; legumes (beans and peas); fruits; vegetables.

Healthy choices. Choose whole grains over refined ones. Choose whole
fruits and vegetables over juice. Buy organic fruits and vegetables and eat
the fiber-rich peel. Sprinkle high-fiber bran cereal or flaxseed on your cereal. Drink lots of water and increase your fiber intake slowly and gradually.

fiber, and just adding a bowl a day has been shown to reduce cholesterol levels. Choose whole fruit and vegetables over juice, which contains almost no fiber.

A teaspoon of psyllium (the generic version of Metamucil) a day will also help you to achieve an additional 2 or 3 percent reduction in cholesterol.

If you increase your fiber gradually and make sure to drink lots of water, your body will become accustomed to the new levels, and you'll be able to sidestep uncomfortable gastrointestinal distress.

USING THE BUILDING BLOCKS TO BUILD A DIET PLAN

So fat, carbohydrates, and protein (with a little information on fiber and cholesterol thrown in for good measure) are the basic building blocks of every healthy diet.

It's how we construct those healthy diets—what percentage of the building blocks goes into each one—that changes everything. If you mix concrete with too much sand or too much water, it won't hold together. That sand/water ratio has to change, depending on temperature, altitude, and a whole host of other factors. The same is true when we're building a diet plan. We have to take all the available factors into account before we can come up with a fat/protein/carbohydrate ratio that's going to address whatever specific underlying metabolic condition we're trying to address.

People are physiologically different, and a standard-issue, die-cut therapy path simply won't work for everyone. Now, with the information contained in your Cardiac Fingerprint, we can prescribe different, individualized therapy paths for everyone. A basic understanding of these building blocks is all you need to follow the program for weight loss and also the Diet Plans that follow!

THE WEIGHT-LOSS PRESCRIPTION

Obesity is the great American albatross. Despite a multibillion-dollar diet industry, we're overweight and unhappy about it, and nothing we do seems to work. In fact, America is getting more and more obese. In the 10 years between the 1980s and early 1990s, there was a 50 percent increase in the number of obese people in the United States. But this issue wouldn't be as fraught with hunger, poor results, and guilt if we stopped choosing fads and weird science over common sense and slow, steady progress.

This discussion of weight loss is designed for those of you—and that will be many!—who need to lose weight, even if it's just a little bit.

In the next section you'll receive an individualized Diet Plan that will ensure you're getting the right nutritional balance of foods to ensure your overall and cardiac health. But the first step in using food to combat coronary heart disease is to make sure that you're at your ideal weight.

I encourage you to read this chapter even if you don't need to lose weight. A therapy path that includes diet isn't about deprivation and weight loss—it's about developing good nutritional habits and adding more delicious, healthful foods to your repertoire. You may be gifted with the metabolism of a jackrabbit, but if you're subsisting entirely on cupcakes and potato chips, you're not much healthier than someone carrying extra weight.

A feature that will be useful to every single one of you, overweight or not, is the tool to help you determine your own caloric needs based on your height, weight, and activity level. One of the first steps in moving away from a one-size-fits-all dietary recommendation is to establish each person's specific caloric needs—the amount of energy fuel *you* need to get through a day. The general recommendations and ballpark figures that prevail throughout the health community are just too general to be helpful. The idea that a single calorie requirement can truly address the needs of two women—a 5-foot 11-inch triathlete and a 5-foot 2-inch couch potato—is patently ridiculous. In this section, I'll give you the information to approximate your own particular calorie needs.

I'll also talk about the reasons that people become overweight and the effects of carrying extra weight on your physiology, especially your heart. And if you're overweight, you'll find a wealth of information, gathered from my experience with my own patients, about healthy, simple ways to change your eating habits and shed those excess pounds.

THE IMPORTANCE OF WEIGHT LOSS

Bill is a 69-year-old overweight diabetic with hypertension, and his cholesterol and metabolic numbers are getting worse and worse. He's already on a list of medications the length of my arm—his primary physician has him taking stuff for his joint pain and his diabetes, and now he's taking niacin, folic acid, and a high–blood pressure medication for me.

He's not showing any signs of cardiac improvement, and I'm getting concerned that he's heading for real trouble. So what are my therapeutic options? I could put him on even more drugs or increase the dosages of the drugs he's already on. It's a risk: He's going to have to accept the additional expense, side effects, and possible drug interactions as well as the very real possibility that more drugs won't work well enough.

Or I could encourage Bill to take a step back and look at the real problem instead of treating its symptoms. The simple truth is that this guy has to lose weight. He's looking to me for answers because I'm the one in the white coat with the prescription pad. But there's nothing I can prescribe for him, no fancy medical wizardry, no sexy science, that would have as great an impact as losing those extra pounds. The most effective prescription I can give Bill is to encourage him to manage his diet and exercise programs so that he'll begin to burn more calories than he consumes, resulting in the loss of his excess body fat.

Losing weight—even as little as 10 pounds!—would be better than all the medication prescriptions I could possibly write for him. It wouldn't cost him a cent, and it's a change that would impact every corner of his health, not just his heart. I'm willing to bet that every single item on that laundry list of complaints would improve dramatically if Bill lost some weight. Yes, it would improve his cardiac health, and we'd rapidly see the difference in his blood pressure and cholesterol numbers. But it would also radically improve his diabetes—a common disease in the overweight. It would help to improve the pain in his joints by relieving them of weight they're not designed to support. And it would make his wife happy. What's the downside—having to shop for new pants?

You wouldn't believe what a dramatic difference weight loss can make. Another one of my patients is an illustrious heart surgeon. The first time I saw him, his numbers were horrifying. I put him on an aggressive course of niacin, but because his schedule was so crazy, he didn't take it consistently, and the numbers kept climbing in the wrong direction. (You'd think a doctor would be better about taking care of himself, but he was typical of many physicians—he couldn't even make the time for his follow-up tests.) Suddenly, a year later, a new set of his numbers came across my desk—and they were fabulous! I called him up, completely thrilled. "I'm so glad you're responding so well to the niacin!" I said. "Uh, actually, the niacin didn't work out," he responded. "I can never remember to take the stuff. I just lost 40 pounds instead."

Ask anyone who works with the heart, and they'll tell you that loss of excess body weight is the *single most important* lifestyle component that can contribute to reduced rates of coronary heart disease.

And yet, as a country, we're getting fatter and fatter. In the past 10 years, there has been a 55 percent increase in the number of people defined as "obese" in the United States. And the greatest increase (about 70 percent!) has been in people between the ages of 18 and 29. This doesn't exactly bode well for America's cardiovascular future. In fact, obesity is such an important issue that the Internal Revenue Service announced in 2002 (ruling 202-19) that since obesity is a medically accepted disease, the expense of treatment is deductible. So if you don't listen to your doctor, maybe you'll listen to the tax man!

I'm not exaggerating when I say that maintaining an appropriate weight is one of the single most powerful tools you have to get the upper hand on the genetic deck that nature dealt you. Isn't it empowering to know that the ability to improve your odds is in your control? And that it's absolutely free and comes with no negative side effects? Don't squander that shot on a chocolate shake!

It Doesn't Have to Be a Lot

One of the big myths about weight loss is that you have to lose a lot to see a difference in your health.

If you're 50 pounds overweight, you don't have to lose 49 to see results. Sure, that's the best-case scenario. But even a 10- or 15-pound loss can have a truly profound effect on your blood test results; every little bit makes a difference. So don't let the magnitude of the project overwhelm you, because you'll start seeing results very early in the process.

So how do you know if you need to lose weight? Some of you have been struggling with weight issues for as long as you can remember. Some of you may have noticed a quiet and insidious spread over the last few years—a belt hole here, a strained button there. Some of you may be genuinely confused by the steroid-enhanced men and emaciated women that dominate in the media—are they a "normal" weight? And if they are, what does that make you?

Help is on the way.

Am I overweight?

Body mass index (BMI) is one of the most widely used methods for determining whether you need to lose weight. In general, if your BMI (see page 34 for a chart that will give you yours) is over 25, you are considered overweight and most likely need to take steps to lose some excess fat. Easier said than done, you may be thinking. While it's true that there's no magic bullet, no overnight fad diet or pill that will make you lose weight and keep it off, the process is actually a lot more straightforward than you might think. It's not magic. All you have to do is educate yourself, do a little planning, and make some lifestyle changes.

Weight Loss and the Diet Plans

In the next section, you'll find a Diet Plan intended specifically for you, and that's going to help you drop down a size or two because it's already designed to take your metabolic sensitivities into account. If too many carbohydrates are making your heart unhealthy, doesn't it follow that your body's inability to handle those carbs would manifest itself in other ways? By getting fat, for instance? Following a diet that's designed for your cardiac type will help you to shed the pounds more easily. And when you combine your individual Diet Plan with your Exercise Prescription, you'll be well on your way to health-promoting weight loss and improving scores on your cholesterol and advanced marker tests.

Be the Animal You're Designed to Be

Weight loss doesn't have to be an exercise in futility. All you have to do is get back to being the animal you were designed to be.

The climbing rate of obesity in America contributes greatly to our epidemic rates of coronary heart disease. If this keeps up, it's predicted that by 2030, a full 50 percent of Americans will be obese. But why are we so fat? We now think that it has to do with a cluster of genes that helps humans to survive in a primitive environment. In 1962, a scientist by the name of Dr. Neel proposed that a cluster of genes must exist to help humans survive in a primitive society, by making us good at holding on to calories and good at moving fats around the body. This is now referred to as the "thrifty gene" concept.

The thrifty gene was a useful trick when we had to hunt for our food. There would be times of great plenty, followed by periods of hunger. When food was available, humans with this trait could stockpile fat and have a better chance of survival than those who could not. Women have more menstrual irregularities below a certain body weight (professional athletes and marathon runners often stop menstruating while they're in training), and since that affects fertility, it was in our bodies' best interests to figure out a way to keep body weight above that point.

So for 500,000 years, we benefited from a genetic structure that favored pigging out. In order to ensure the survival of the species, our bodies got really good at storing up calories after the feasts so that we wouldn't starve during the leaner times. If you ate as much food as possible when it was available, you stood a better chance of surviving, looking good to the opposite sex, and successfully procreating than those who didn't. This is all fine and good if you're living in an environment where your food supply may be compromised in the 2 days after your binge, but in the past 200 years, many human societies have had the opposite problem: an abundance of calories.

When you eat too many calories, this genetic attribute may kick in. Of course, our ancestors were doing hard physical labor, and they'd use the calories they'd stored while waiting for the results of the next successful hunt. Exercise and going hungry allow this genetic trait to do what it was designed to do and help us survive. But for most Americans, there's not a lot of hard physical labor, and few starving times—our food supply is not only plentiful and inexpensive, but extraordinarily calorie rich. And so that survival gene turns into a deadly one.

What we have is a gene-environment mismatch: When that gene cluster is active and we greedily consume every calorie laid before us even though it's no longer necessary for our survival, we create a metabolic condition that's very harmful for our hearts. In fact, since overweight is so closely linked to coronary heart disease and diabetes, this thrifty gene is really working against our better interests these days. You can actually make the argument that the coronary heart disease is an outcome of the success of the human species in acquiring an abundant food supply!

This thrifty gene concept provides us with a rational explanation for why you have to exercise an hour a day, 7 days a week—you have to turn yourself into the animal that you're designed to be. But more on that later. Let's focus first on weight loss through a proper diet.

Know What You're Eating

Learning to eat so that you lose weight may require that you educate yourself a little. Women in America tend to be more (and often unhealthily) concerned about their weight than men, so they're often better educated about the calories and fat in common foods. Men, on the other hand, are often completely oblivious about what foods they're putting in their mouths.

For instance, did you know that one of those "blooming onion" appetizers at the neighborhood joint where you stop for a drink on Friday nights contains more than 3 *days'* worth of saturated fat? And well over the number of calories you should consume in the whole day, with little nutritional value at all to show for it? And you thought it was just something to snack on over a beer.

Think about it this way: You burn about 100 calories with every mile you walk briskly. That means that you have to walk 2 miles to get rid of that chocolate chip cookie you popped into your mouth without a second thought during a catered meeting. Six miles to make a dent in the fast-food burger that you picked up at the drive-in because you were too tired to cook. And we're not even talking yet about the amount—and type—of fat in those meals.

Even some of the things we think are good for us are hiding a scary number of calories. A salad's health food, right? But with Caesar dressing, you're looking at 3½ miles. Olive oil is full of those heart-healthy monounsaturated fats, but it's also 100 calories a tablespoon, and you can sop up a tablespoon pretty easily with a single piece of yummy Italian bread. Have a big deli-style bagel for breakfast, and you're already up to 4 miles before you've even added the cream cheese or the butter.

But all food's not created equal. You'd have to eat 6½ apples to equal the calorie load of that unbuttered bagel. You could eat two whole tomatoes in the place of that tablespoon of oil. And you could burn off an entire bag of lettuce greens just walking around your house. That's a lot of food! So you have a lot of control over how much you eat and how full you get just by making healthy choices.

How many calories do you need?

Conventional wisdom has it that most men can lose weight on a diet that provides them with about 1,800 calories a day, and most women can lose weight on a diet that provides them with about 1,200 a day.

Since we're moving away from a single, monolithic treatment theory in all the other areas of this book, why would weight loss be any different? Obviously, a man who's 6'2" and 210 pounds of solid, active muscle has different calorie requirements than one who's 5'7" and sits behind a desk all day. There's a much more specific way to figure out how many calories you need to survive in any given day, and how many you have to cut to lose weight at a sensible and healthy rate.

We all burn calories just by existing. In other words, if you never got out of bed at all, you'd still burn a certain number of calories. That's called your basal metabolic rate (BMR). You need that number of calories simply to survive. You can figure out your own BMR using the Harris-Benedict Equations.

Men	Women
66	655
+ (13.7 × weight in kilograms)	+ (9.6 × weight in kilograms)
+ (5 × height in centimeters)	+ (1.8 × height in centimeters)
− (6.8 × age in years)	− (4.7 × age in years)
BMR=	BMR=

Get a calculator, and let's take it step by step. These equations are in metric, so most Americans will need this conversion information.

Your weight in kilograms is your weight in pounds divided by 2.2. So if you weigh 180 pounds, we divide that number by 2.2 to get 81.8 kilograms.

Your height in centimeters is your height in inches multiplied by 2.54. If you're 5'7" tall, you're 67 inches. 67 inches multiplied by 2.54 is 170.18 centimeters. So a 5'7" man is 170 centimeters tall.

The BMR for Tom, a 54-year-old man (who just happens to be 5'7" tall and 180 pounds) would be:

$$BMR = 66 + (13.7 \times 81.8) + (5 \times 170) - (6.8 \times 54) = 1{,}669.5 \text{ calories.}$$

Now, your BMR is a slightly rough tool: Someone who's more muscular will burn more than someone who's unfit. But this provides you with a very good starting guideline.

And of course, nobody stays in bed all day—even if your daily exercise isn't more than light activity, you're burning more than your BMR as soon as you put your feet into your slippers in the morning.

This activity multiplier will help you to discover approximately how many calories you're *actually* burning every day.

Sedentary (little or no exercise, desk job) = BMR × 1.2
Lightly active (light exercise 1 to 3 days a week) = BMR × 1.375
Moderately active (moderate exercise 3 to 5 days a week) = BMR × 1.55
Very active (hard exercise 6 or 7 days a week) = BMR × 1.725
Superactive (hard daily exercise and hard physical job) = BMR × 1.9

Now Tom's what you might call sedentary—he walks from the house to the car to the office to the car to the house, and that's pretty much it. His BMR was 1,670 calories, but he's actually burning (slightly) more than that: 1,670 × 1.2, which is the activity level for a sedentary person. 1,670 × 1.2 = 2,004 calories. So Tom actually needs about 2,000 calories to get through a given day.

If you've done your own calculations, you'll know what you're burning every day. That's an essential piece of information, because you must run a calorie deficit to lose weight. It's like balancing a budget. If you make more than you spend, your balance will increase. If you burn more calories than you take in, you will lose weight.

Now let's find out how many calories you're actually taking in.

Keep a Food Record

One of the most important steps in losing weight is learning to be more aware of what you eat. I've discovered that a lot of my patients, especially the busy ones, don't even know what they're eating. They shovel a sandwich in between phone calls, they order a couple of desserts for the table at dinner, they feast late-night with the refrigerator door open. To combat this, I often ask my patients to keep a food journal, in which they record everything they eat and drink for 3 days.

I'd like you to keep a food record for 3 days as well. It won't be too much of a burden to you, and I think you'll find it very informative. Just eat normally, and write down what you eat. You don't have to weigh your food or anything crazy, although I would like you to keep a general record of portion size ("a hamburger patty the size of my fist" or "a cookie the size of a coaster"). Don't cheat—write down everything you eat, even snacks grabbed on the run ("half of a cookie the size of a coaster") and everything you drink—even water. Make a note of the times you eat these items as well.

Keeping this record will be useful in a number of ways. First of all, when you review the final results, you'll be able to see what you're eating. You can isolate healthy and unhealthy patterns, and that will help you to make healthy changes to your diet. Replace that afternoon pastry with low-sodium pretzels and a piece of fruit, for instance, or substitute turkey for pastrami, and you'll see a significant savings in calories and fat. Also, you'll gather important information about when you tend to overeat. Do you tend to raid the leftovers when the house is dark, or is that low-blood-sugar trap every afternoon at 4:00 driving you to the vending machine? Are you blowing the benefits of your healthy choices with gigantic portions? Are you skipping breakfast and making up for it in spades at lunch?

Keeping the journal will also make you more conscious of the bad food habits you may have without realizing it. Did you know that you had a doughnut *every* afternoon, or do you still think of it as a once-in-a-while treat? So many of us snack thoughtlessly—it's the downside of living in a country where food is so plentiful. And keeping the journal will make you accountable for what you eat *before* you eat it: You're less likely to reach for the cookie you don't really even want if you know you're going to have to record it in black and white.

This lesson came home to roost in a very personal way for me a couple of years ago. I suddenly realized that I'd put on about 6 pounds, and I couldn't figure out where it had come from. I didn't feel like I was eating any more than usual (and I can assure you, this wasn't 6 pounds of muscle). So I kept a food record for a couple of days and nabbed the culprit: the oatmeal-raisin cookie I'd made the habit of picking up along with my lunch every day. It never occurred to me that it was a big deal—an innocent cookie, and "healthy" oatmeal, too!—but it was a big enough deal to move me up a belt hole. So now it really is just a special treat.

Lastly, this document is going to provide an important benchmark of your eating habits before you went on the Diet Plan. In the next section, you'll see what you *should* be eating, given your inherited attributes and underlying cardiac conditions, and you'll be able to compare it to what you've been eating up to this point. When you're looking for food items in your record to cut out and substitute with healthier choices, you'll be able to look at your diet with a much-better-educated eye. Want to know why your cholesterol level hasn't budged, despite your best efforts? Want to know why your weight-loss efforts have continually been thwarted? Hopefully, we're setting you up for an "a-ha!" moment here.

> Calories required to survive + extra calories = FAT!

If you need to lose weight, you're going to have to determine how many calories you're taking in on a regular basis, using your food journal. The easiest way to go about this is to keep track as you go along, but you can also do it at the end of the day. Food manufacturers are obligated to list calorie information on the packaging, there are any number of calorie counters at your bookstore, and there are a million free sites on the Internet with calorie information. Be honest and make sure you're taking portion size into account. Keep this calorie log for a couple of days and you'll start to get a general idea of what you're averaging.

Once you have that average, you have the crucial information you need to determine the discrepancy between what you need to eat and what you're actually eating.

If you close that gap, you will lose weight.

Let's look at an example. We've determined that Tom, the 54-year-old in the BMR example on page 143, needs about 1,670 calories a day just to survive. And he's pretty sedentary, so we'll say he needs 2,000 calories to get through his day. Then we take a look at his food journal and discover that he's been eating about 2,700 calories a day. With no further ado, the mystery of his bulging waistline has been solved.

The good news is that—and you should forgive the pun—there's a lot of fat to be trimmed in his caloric intake. 2,700 calories is a lot of calories, and he's wasting a lot of them on junk—calories that add up without filling you up. If he replaces some of his habitual splurges with healthier choices (in other words, decreases the number of calories he eats) and begins a daily exercise program (increasing the number of calories he burns), he'll be able to cut 500 calories a day, which will add up to about a pound of fat a week.

If 500 calories a day is too much to cut from your diet alone and you find yourself hungry, make it 300 for the first little while and get that extra 200 calories from your exercise program. Concentrate on improving the quality of the food you're eating while your body adjusts. Interestingly, although it seems counterintuitive, increased physical activity is often associated with reduced hunger. Ask your friends who exercise regularly, and they'll tell you that a good workout helps them to control their appetite!

Weight-Loss Tips

Since weight loss is such a crucial component of this program, I get lots of feedback from my patients on what works for them and what doesn't. I'd like to share some of their hard-won experience with you.

Snack smart. As everyone who's ever found herself eating a bag of marshmallows at 2:00 A.M. knows, if there's nothing healthy in the house, you're going to eat what's there. Keep healthy snacks around and accessible. Vegetables should be cut and peeled and ready to grab in a Tupperware container on the top shelf. Put fruit in a bowl on the counter so you see it right away. Get rid of the junk that tempts you!

Look ahead. Shopping is a crucial step, and you need to know what you're going to be eating over the course of the week so you can shop in advance. Even if you're not the main chef of the house, act as consultant. And don't go shopping when you're hungry. You should be pushing the cart, not your thrifty gene.

Start small. Small changes can make a big difference. Choose a salad over fries, and with that small decision, you've already cut most of the calories you need to eliminate in a given day.

Don't deprive yourself. If you forbid yourself to have any of the stuff you love, you're not going to be able to stick with your new eating plan. Indulge every once in a while, and pick up the slack with something you don't feel as passionately about. A square of chocolate or a bite of something sinful once a week isn't going to kill you, and you won't feel deprived if you have a little. Just don't eat a full portion of it, and don't eat it every day.

Eat frequent, small meals. You don't have to be hungry to lose weight— in fact, it's a bad idea. We all overeat if we let ourselves get too hungry. Don't hesitate to eat a healthy snack if you're hungry an hour before dinner. You'll be less likely to wolf it down like a maniac if you're not starving when it's served. Eat a healthy snack before a party. If you're already full, you won't need to stalk the waiter with the crab canapes. You can eat lots of food as long as you're eating healthy food—and not too much of it.

Try the carrot trick. I often suggest to my patients that they keep a container of raw, peeled carrots in the refrigerator (the bags of baby carrots that are so widely available work well). I make them a deal: They can have an unhealthy snack as long as they have a carrot (or six of the baby ones) first. It's like magic! Eating the carrot often completely removes the desire for that unhealthy snack.

Prepare your food wisely. That vegetable stir-fry is a delicious and healthy dinner, but not if you dump a cup of oil in the wok to get things started—at 100 calories a tablespoon, you'll find yourself in Big Mac territory pretty fast despite your best efforts. Use oil sparingly, and substitute chicken broth or water if you need a little liquid to make sure things don't stick.

Slow down. It takes about 20 minutes for your stomach to send the message to your brain that it's well-fed. The more slowly you eat, the less you'll have consumed by the time you get full. Wait 20 minutes after your first helping to determine that you're still hungry enough for seconds. More often than not, that second plate of food won't appeal.

Watch portion sizes. As everything's gotten supersized, we seem to have lost our perspective on a normal-size portion of food. A cup, which is roughly the size of your closed fist, is a standard portion for a bowl of cereal—not that swimming pool–size bowl you've been using. The standard portion for a piece of meat is 3 to 4 ounces—the size of a deck of cards. A normal portion of cheese is a single ounce: a 1-inch by 1-inch cube. Look at your food record—how far off the mark are you? Start paying attention to your portion sizes of the high-calorie stuff, and fill the rest of the plate with vegetables, salad, and fruit.

Don't crash diet. A healthy weight loss is approximately a pound a week—no more. Starving yourself is unhealthy and unwise. First of all, you won't take the weight off. If your body senses it's being starved, it'll go into defensive mode and you'll start hoarding calories. Statistically speaking, people who lose weight slowly and gradually by changing their eating habits and developing an exercise program are the people who keep the weight off.

Exercise regularly. As we'll discuss in the Exercise Prescription, exercising burns calories. It burns them while you're exercising, it continues to burn them for hours after you stop, and it helps you to build muscle, which increases your basal metabolic rate—in other words, a muscular person burns more calories just sitting around than a fat one does. Exercise also alters how efficiently your body metabolizes food, which naturally contributes to weight loss. Plus, people who exercise regularly are less likely to overeat, and people who lose weight through exercise are more likely to keep it off.

Watch what you drink. A soda at lunch adds 150 calories; a glass of wine at dinner adds another 150, and they don't do anything to make you less hungry. Forget the economy-size soda at the movies—it's not a better deal if it's packing on another 150 calories. Getting those calories back is as easy as substituting a glass of water (or diet soda, or soda water) for one of those drinks.

Eat Out Smart

Sure, it's easy to eat healthily if you're in a hermetically sealed bubble where you control all of your own shopping and meal decisions and cooking methods. But the real world isn't like that. In the real world, we grab a sandwich and some chips at a catered meeting; we're wined and dined on expense accounts; we find ourselves starving in a hotel room at midnight with nothing but a limited room-service menu for consolation, or the snack machine down the hall.

A lot of us think of restaurants as "treats" and therefore diet-free zones, although we eat out a number of times a week! Fat tastes good, so restaurants use a lot of it to keep us coming back, but it is possible to eat healthily when we're eating out. For all of this diet advice to actually work, it has to fit into your real-world lifestyle. You're going to have to learn to eat out smarter.

Here are some tricks.

Choose healthy protein. Choosing fish and white-meat poultry (breast meat, as opposed to leg or thigh) over red meat is always a safe bet. You can radically reduce the calories in your chicken or turkey dish just by removing the skin. At a deli, low-fat tuna salad is a much better choice than the full-fat kind; turkey breast is even better. Hold the mayo and choose seven-grain bread instead of white toast.

Pay attention to preparation. Look at the way food is prepared: Words like "grilled," "steamed," "broiled" are good. "Fried" and "sautéed" usually mean that a dish has been prepared with a lot of oil.

Ask. Don't be afraid to ask questions about the ingredients and the way a dish is prepared, and don't be afraid to make special requests. Restaurants are used to making accommodations for people with special dietary needs. You're not the first person to ask them to leave the cheese off the top.

Fast food doesn't have to be fat food. It's not your healthiest choice (fast food tends to be high in sodium and low in fiber), but the drive-through doesn't necessarily have to mean the death of your diet. The counter person can provide you with a list of nutritional information; take the time to look at your options and make healthy choices. The same thing goes here as in other restaurants: Let common sense prevail. The iceberg lettuce fast-food places tend to use is hardly ideal, but a grilled chicken sandwich (hold the mayo) with a side salad is still a better option than a supersized triple-decker burger with sauce and a side of fries, which contains more than a full day's calorie load and a week's worth of saturated fat.

Watch out for side dishes. Those mashed potatoes are just butter and heavy cream with some spuds thrown in for good measure. Most restaurants are happy to replace unhealthy sides like french fries with a salad. If they won't, ask them to leave the item off altogether and order a side salad instead.

Don't drink your meal. A drink before dinner, half a bottle of wine, and a glass of port afterward contain all the calories you need to consume at one meal, with absolutely no nutritional value or satiety attached. Make sure you've figured liquor into your calorie allowance if you choose to drink it. And remember that liquor lowers inhibitions, which means that it can impair your plan to eat in moderation.

Master dessert. Most menus offer a "healthy" choice dessert, like cut fresh fruit or a selection of sorbets. If the others at your table want to share the "Death by Chocolate" and you can't resist it, take a bite and then put your fork down.

To splurge or not to splurge?

One of the questions I hear most often from my patients is whether or not it's all right to splurge on a high-fat meal every once in a while. Of course it is. A sugar doughnut once a month isn't going to give you a heart attack—I certainly indulge every once in a while. The only exception I can think of is if your triglycerides are high. A high-fat meal can really blow your triglycerides out of the water, and if you're someone who struggles with high triglycerides ordinarily, that kind of jump can increase triglycerides to the point where they impair your blood's ability to deliver oxygen to your muscles—muscles like your heart. I'd settle for a single bite or two of the tempting food.

I counsel all my patients against extended splurges. A lot of my patients see a resurgence of their dormant angina on their vacations. A high-fat meal is one thing; a 2-week calorie and fat splurge while you're on a cruise is another thing entirely. When my patients ask how much leeway they can have on their vacations, I always tell them this story: A number of years ago, a research group did a clinical trial on two groups of monkeys with atherosclerosis, which was given to both groups through a high-fat diet. One group stayed on the high-fat foods while the other was put on a strictly controlled low-fat diet. Unsurprisingly, at the end of a couple of years, the disease in the monkeys in the low-fat group looked much better than it did in the other group.

Then the researchers did something smart: They let the low-fat monkeys pig out on a high-fat diet for a couple of weeks. At the end of that short period, they discovered that the low-fat monkeys had lost *all* of their gains— their hearts looked like those of the monkeys who had been on the high-fat diet all along. The same artery plaques that had taken 2 years to shrink down on the low-fat diet swelled back up after only 2 weeks on a high-fat diet. So the results of 2 years of "being good" were completely wiped out by a couple of weeks of gluttony.

Now, monkeys aren't people, but this is as good as the clinical testing is going to get since this isn't the kind of study you could ethically do in humans. I personally think this monkey study is a pretty strong argument against restaging the dinner scene from Fellini's *Satyricon* on your vacation. If you develop good nutritional habits, then you won't get into trouble when you're faced with temptation. In this chapter, we hope to give you the tools to choose heart-healthy foods no matter where you are.

Watch out, in particular, at the holidays. There's a phenomenon known in cardiology circles as "the matzo ball syndrome." Matzo ball soup is a common addition to dinner at Passover, one of the Jewish holidays. Although it looks harmless enough—unleavened cracker-dough balls in a chicken broth—it's loaded with sodium and sends hypertensive celebrants to hospitals in droves with congestive heart failure.

So don't let your mother needle you into second helpings, and ask how food is prepared, the same way you would in a restaurant. Your loved ones won't mind—they want to keep you healthy too.

Reaching and maintaining a healthy weight is part of the first Prescription because it's the first, essential step toward cardiac health. Now, as we continue on through the Nutrition Prescription, we'll be looking at ways to treat your metabolic conditions through *what* you eat.

THE DIET PLANS

Here's a scenario that happens all too often.

Jim's doctor tells him that his cholesterol is high and advises him to begin a low-fat diet. They agree to a follow-up appointment in 3 months. In 3 months, Jim's numbers haven't improved, so Jim's doctor recommends that he go on medication. Jim takes the drugs, drops the diet, and his worrisome cholesterol numbers improve.

Jim now believes that he's a diet nonresponder—someone for whom diet doesn't work to improve the underlying factors that put him at risk for coronary heart disease. And he'll be on medication for the rest of his life.

But what if Jim *isn't* a nonresponder? What if he was just on the wrong diet? What if he could use his three squares a day as medication—instead of that expensive drug with all its side-effect risks and compliance requirements?

With a little additional information—information that *you* now have in your Cardiac Fingerprint—Jim could have seen very different results at that 3-month checkup. I believe that if Jim's doctor had been able to "prescribe" something better than the standard-issue, low-fat diet, a diet specifically oriented to Jim's genetic makeup and underlying conditions, they would both have been rewarded by greatly improved numbers.

I want to bring the latest research out of the laboratory, out of your cardiologist's examining room, and right onto your dinner table.

A number of the metabolic conditions that cause coronary heart disease can be affected by what you eat and in what percentage. That's right: You can actually make changes at the metabolic level that directly affect your coronary heart disease risk by changing the percentage of those basic nutritional building blocks we talked about earlier. Diet, once it is truly customized to your cardiac profile, is a very powerful tool, even replacing the need for medication in certain cases. It may not replace medication for all of you, but whether it's used alone or in combination with a drug therapy, the right diet will certainly have a profound effect on your ability to cheat your genetic predisposition toward coronary heart disease.

CHOOSE WHOLE FOODS

No matter which of the three Diet Plans in my Nutrition Prescription ends up being the right diet for your particular metabolic type, you'll find that they all emphasize whole, nutrient-dense, unprocessed grains, fruits, and vegetables. This is a healthy recommendation for *every* heart.

It seems that when you get into cardiac trouble, one of the first things that your doctor will tell you to do is to go on a low-fat diet, and even people who don't have problems with their hearts worry about their fat intake. In my opinion, the single-minded focus on fat in all the dietary discussions on heart health has made Americans myopic on the issue. We're cramming ourselves full of fake, sugar-laden foods just because their labels trumpet that they're fat-free.

But we're missing an essential piece of the puzzle. The evidence is incontrovertible: People who eat more fruits and vegetables have less coronary heart disease—and less cancer. Whole foods—fruits, vegetables, legumes, whole grains—are low-fat or fat-free, but unlike those fake foods, they come with a host of other benefits. They're fiber rich, which helps regulate cholesterol and reduces risk of coronary heart disease. They tend to be low on the glycemic index, so they naturally help to regulate our blood sugar and energy level. They're packed with protective antioxidants—those we know about, like vitamin C, beta-carotene, and vitamin E—and those whose beneficial effects we haven't yet discovered.

We've been swinging wildly from one extreme dietary measure to the next, when the answer has been in front of us all the time: Eat moderate amounts of whole, real foods.

AVOID SATURATED FAT

Just because I think we have to get away from our fat-free lockstep doesn't mean that I'm blithely counseling you to sit down to a dinner-size plate of foie gras. If a "normal meal" at a fast-food restaurant can contain a few days'—days'!—worth of saturated fats, something about the way we think about this issue of fat is seriously out of whack. I'm simply concerned that this concentration of our attention on fat comes at the expense of the rest of our diet: No-fat cookies made entirely of sugars aren't the answer to our problems either! You'll see that all three of the diets in my Nutrition Prescription steer you away from saturated fat, no matter what your metabolic profile is.

HEALTHY CHOICES: CUTTING FAT

What are the best ways to cut fat, especially the saturated kind?

- Eat red meat much less often, and cut the portion size of all the meat you eat. *A meat portion (3 ounces) is the size of a deck of cards.*

- Cut your added fats: the butter, the margarine, and the oils you add to salad dressings and use in cooking.

   I often tell my patients: "If you do nothing else, do these two things, and I guarantee that we'll see a reduction in your weight and LDL-C." And we do, so it's advice worth passing on.

Unlike many cardiologists, I don't believe that a low-fat, high-carbohydrate diet is automatically the right prescription for every cardiac patient. In the Diet Plans that follow, you'll see that I recommend a lower-fat diet for some people and a higher-fat diet for others—but that all of them restrict *saturated* fats. Although I'm much more lenient in general about fat than many cardiologists, I'm actually much stricter about saturated fat, because those fats have the greatest impact on lipid levels. The American Heart Association's recommendation is to restrict saturated fat to 10 percent of total calories; none of my Diet Plans go above 6 percent. We have to educate ourselves about the different kinds of fat and learn to cut saturated fats and use monounsaturated fats in their place. These three Diet Plans necessarily emphasize low-fat protein sources, such as egg whites, soy products, lean cuts of meat, white-meat poultry, and low-fat or fat-free dairy. And they all derive essential fatty acids from fish, canola, and olive oil.

In this chapter, I hope to paint a much healthier vision of the way you can put fat into its proper place in your diet without sacrificing taste—or your health.

BLOOD PRESSURE AND DIET

As we know, high blood pressure is a serious risk factor contributing to coronary heart disease, and for a long time, we believed that sodium—salt—was the villain of that particular set piece. Certainly, a high-sodium diet does play a role in hypertension, and some people are particularly responsive to a low-sodium diet. But a new set of clinical trials called DASH (Dietary Approaches to Stop Hypertension) gives us more guidelines to address blood pressure through dietary measures.

The DASH diet is rich in fruits and vegetables, fat-free or low-fat dairy products, whole grains, fish, poultry, and nuts. It reduces the amount of red meat and sweets. It is high in fiber, low in sodium, and includes minerals that we know contribute to lowered blood pressure, such as calcium, magnesium, and potassium.

All three of the Diet Plans that follow were designed to fit within the parameters of the DASH diet.

WEIGHT LOSS AND THE NUTRITION PRESCRIPTION

All the diet recommendations and menu plans here are based on a 2,000-calorie diet, which is considered to be a maintenance calorie load, the number of calories that the average man requires in a given day. For some of you, this won't work, either because you're not "average" or because you're not men!

As you will see throughout this book, I'm trying to get us away from the one-size-fits-all school of thought, and that extends to the number of calories you consume. It's ridiculous to assume that different people of different sizes, gender, and activity levels will need the same number of calories over the course of a given day. That's why we provided the equations to figure out your approximate daily calorie load in the previous section on weight loss. If you haven't already done that math, you'll want to go back to page 143 and do it so that you can alter the Diet Plan accordingly to accommodate your caloric requirements.

In most cases, you'll easily be able to make up the difference. Each of the snacks recommended in the Diet Plans comes to about 200 calories. By cutting those and increasing your exercise by 300 calories a day, you'll cut the 500 daily calories needed to lose a pound a week. If you know that you need to eat more than 2,000 calories a day, you can simply make up the difference by adding a healthy snack or small meal—within the parameters of your Diet Plan, of course.

ONE STEP AT A TIME

The way we eat is fundamental to who we are, and changes to our familiar routine often feel overwhelming. The way you eat has taken a lifetime to develop, and you're going to have to change it one step at a time. I recommend that my patients make changes to their diets gradually. Rome wasn't built in a day, and you won't fix the diet part of your lipid problem overnight.

In my practice, I've found that people often do best with the things that are familiar to them. For instance, recipes that you grew up with can usually be modified to reflect your new eating pattern. Prioritize your changes. Which changes will have the most impact on your numbers? Which changes will be the easiest to make? Find the balance between the two and start there. And if something's not working, approach it from another angle.

Most importantly, you have to have patience with yourself. This isn't an all-or-nothing process—you're changing the way you eat for life. If you have a devil-may-care weekend, get back up and do better on Monday. It will get easier, I promise. And one day you'll look back at your old food record—and your old marker numbers—in disbelief.

FINDING YOUR NUTRITION PRESCRIPTION

As with the Exercise, Medication, and Supplement components of this program, you'll use the Prescription Key on page 160 to help you locate the individualized Diet Plan that has been calibrated to meet the needs of your particular cardiac profile. All you'll need to do is to match the results of your own tests against the Prescription Key to find the plan that is right for you.

The first Diet Plan is the **Whole Heart Diet**, which uses a balanced combination of whole foods. It's tailored for people who are LDL pattern A and want to stay that way, and for those of you who have a combination of metabolic issues that would benefit from a balanced approach. It's also the place to start if you haven't taken the Advanced Metabolic Marker tests and don't yet have a complete Cardiac Fingerprint with information about your metabolic issues, or as a general recommendation for anyone who's looking to prevent coronary heart disease through diet. The next Diet Plan is the **More-Fat, Low-Fat Diet** (not a low-fat diet, you'll notice!) for the real diet responders out there: people with LDL pattern B, high apo B, and/or apo E4. We've put some of the fat back into the low-fat diet to make it both healthier and tastier for you. And the third plan is the **Better-Carbohydrate, Lower-Carbohydrate**

Diet, for people who exhibit any of the prediabetic issues like chronically high triglycerides or elevated insulin levels.

Using the Prescription Key

Directly below the Nutrition Prescription Key on page 160 you'll see a list of four markers labeled "My Diet Markers." These will determine which individualized Diet Plan is the right fit for your cardiac profile.

Refer to your Quick Reference Chart on page 91 to help you to fill in a "yes" or "no" in the space provided beside each Diet Marker. (Let's do an example together: Mark has tested "abnormal" on LDL pattern B, apo E4, apo B, and insulin, so his column would read "Yes," "Yes," "Yes," and "Yes.")

Once you have your list of yeses and no's, just look up at the Key and find the column that duplicates your pattern. (Remember, read down the columns, from top to bottom, until you find your exact match.)

At the base of the column that matches your own results, you'll find the number that identifies *your* plan! (Mark would find the plan that matches *his* four yeses in the eighth column from the left. Since the number at the base of the column is 3, he should proceed to the third Diet Plan, the Better-Carbohydrate, Lower-Carbohydrate Diet.)

So refer to your Quick Reference Chart on page 91, and let's get started!

Note: If you haven't taken the Advanced Metabolic Marker tests or if you're still waiting for your results, don't worry—we're not leaving you out. You should proceed directly to the first plan, the Whole Heart Diet. When your results come back (or if you decide to be tested in the future), you'll be able to insert your results into the Prescription Key as we've described above.

The Nutrition Prescription Key

Diet Marker																
LDL pattern B	Yes	Yes	Yes	Yes	Yes	Yes	Yes	Yes	No	No	No	No	No	No	No	No
Apo E4	No	Yes	Yes	No	No	Yes	No	No	Yes	Yes	Yes	No	Yes	No	Yes	No
Apo B	No	No	Yes	Yes	Yes	No	Yes	Yes	Yes	No	No	No	Yes	Yes	No	No
Insulin	No	No	No	No	Yes	Yes	Yes	Yes	Yes	No	No	No	No	No	No	No
Diet Plan #:	3	1	2	2	1	1	3	3	1	1	3	1	1	2	1	2

Diet Plan #1: The Whole Heart Diet

Diet Plan #2: The More-Fat, Low-Fat Diet

Diet Plan #3: The Better-Carbohydrate, Lower-Carbohydrate Diet

---

My Diet Markers:

LDL pattern B _____

Apo E4 _____

Apo B _____

Insulin _____

DIET PLAN #1
THE WHOLE HEART DIET

If the best offense is a strong defense, adopting this Diet Plan is a truly aggressive move against coronary heart disease. What are the elements that make this plan such a valuable defense mechanism against coronary heart disease?

- You can immunize yourself against cardiac disease with a Diet Plan calibrated to act as a shield for your cardiovascular system.
- Balance is the key word here, as the benefits of a well-balanced diet extend far beyond the health of your heart.
- Real food—fruits, vegetables, complex carbohydrates, and low-fat protein sources—are your best line of nutritional defense against cardiac risk.

Immunize Yourself!

You can build your immunity to infectious diseases, and you can build your immunity to coronary heart disease, too. Think of the Whole Heart Diet as your diet for cardiac defense, the diet that will help you to make sure that your heart is in the best fighting shape possible.

Today you're not in the danger zone or even close. You might, in fact, have a squeaky clean bill of health—but the point is to make sure it stays that way! Even if you're blessed with pristine genes, a lifetime of saturated fat, supersized portions, and sugary drinks can destroy your natural immunity to coronary heart disease. This diet bolsters and reinforces your heart health so that if you're forced to go into battle against coronary heart disease, your troops are already at a state of high readiness and alert.

Nutrition is one of the best shields you have at your disposal to protect yourself from cardiac disease, and it should be your first line of defense.

Balance

We want to protect our hearts, so we starve our bodies of fat. We want to lose weight, so we eat nothing but protein and trick our bodies into thinking we're starving.

HOW ANTIOXIDANTS PROTECT YOUR HEART

As you'll recall from our discussion of oxidation, the process is a bit like rusting. Antioxidants help keep you from "rusting" on the cellular level. It's like applying a special lubricant to your child's bike chain. Certain foods are rich in antioxidants, and you can help protect yourself against the rusting process simply by eating these foods.

LDL, the "bad" cholesterol, becomes even more dangerous once it is oxidized. When LDL is oxidized, it becomes really desirable bait for the white blood cells that are working to repair the damaged artery walls. In an attempt to protect the body, the white blood cells eat lots of these oxidized LDL particles in the arterial walls, where they cause even more damage. So any Diet Plan that boosts your antioxidants may help to impede the oxidation of LDL, which may slow or even prevent atherosclerosis.

Vitamin C (ascorbic acid), vitamin E (alphatocopherol), and beta-carotene are among the antioxidants that have this effect, and they're all available from dietary sources.

• Good sources of vitamin E include sunflower seeds, almonds, hazelnuts, and wheat germ. Be careful: These sources tend to be high in fats.

• Good sources of vitamin C include strawberries, citrus fruits like grapefruit and oranges, tomatoes, and broccoli.

• Good sources of beta-carotene include sweet potatoes, apricots, peaches, carrots, cantaloupe, squash, and spinach. Beta-carotene is a precursor to vitamin A. As you see, it tends to be found in orange-colored foods.

Eating foods rich in these antioxidants is recommended for everyone. We'll discuss other ways to increase your antioxidant intake in the Supplement Prescription.

So much of what's wrong with the way we eat has to do with this failure to understand the importance of balance! Our grandmothers would call this Whole Heart Diet a "sensible" diet, and they'd be right—it *is* a sensible diet, with a little cutting-edge science thrown in for good measure. (The rate of obesity and coronary heart disease was considerably lower in your grandmother's day, incidentally.)

A low-fat diet is the standard prescription for people with cardiac problems. But if you're one of the people who's unsuccessfully struggled to lower your cholesterol on a very-low-fat diet, here's a shocker for you: In some cases, those low-fat diets may actually be *causing* your cardiac risk factor problems. That's right—the so-called solution is actually contributing to the problem. Swing the pendulum the other way, and you find people eating high-protein diets overloaded with saturated fats. Both extremes are problematic, and both are extremely popular diets today. And Americans wonder why our rates of coronary heart disease are as high as they are!

Let's put some of the common sense and enjoyment back into the way we eat, and our hearts will benefit as a result.

Real Food

As the title of this Diet Plan implies, I'm dedicated to taking the single-minded focus off fad-driven nutritional distractions and putting it back where it belongs: on healthy, whole foods put together in combinations that benefit the whole heart—and the rest of the body as well.

Your body uses food as fuel and as a source of the life-giving vitamins, nutrients, and antioxidants it can't produce. The better the fuel you give it, the better it will run. This diet combines all of our nutritional building blocks in the way that's most likely to work *with* your body rather than against it.

Who Should Use This Diet Plan?

- People with LDL pattern A
- People with multiple metabolic problems
- People who don't yet have a complete Cardiac Fingerprint, but who wish to prevent coronary heart disease

(continued on page 167)

THE FOOD EXCHANGE GUIDE

This food exchange guide will be your tool for devising endlessly varied meals while staying within the guidelines of your prescribed Diet Plan.

Within each Diet Plan, we've provided you with 1 full week of sample menu plans to help get you started. These sample menus are there to give you some ideas and to help you get the hang of your new diet. Here, we've provided you with basic exchanges for each of the food groups, so that you'll be able to freely pick and choose according to your personal preferences. This will enable you to come up with an infinite variety of menu plans of your own.

You'll also find specialized Daily Exchange guides within your individualized Diet Plan. These will provide further support as you try your hand at customizing your own menus.

BREAD, CEREALS, AND STARCHY VEGETABLES

(1 bread/cereal/starchy vegetable exchange or 1 serving = 15 grams of carbohydrate, 3 grams of protein, a trace of fat, and 80 calories)

1 slice whole grain bread

¾ cup ready-to-eat, unsweetened, whole grain cereal

½ cup cooked pasta

⅓ cup cooked brown, brown basmati, or wild rice

½ whole grain bagel

½ whole grain English muffin

½ whole grain hamburger or hot-dog bun

1 corn tortilla (6") or whole wheat tortilla (8")

½ whole wheat pita (6")

1 small whole grain dinner roll

1 small baked potato (3 ounces)

½ cup cooked corn

½ cup lima beans

½ cup green peas

1 cup winter squash

½ cup sweet potato

½ cup orzo

1 cup tomato or vegetable soup

⅓ cup hummus (1 starch + 1 fat)

NONSTARCHY VEGETABLES

(1 nonstarchy vegetable exchange or 1 serving = 5 grams of carbohydrate, 2 grams of protein, 0 fat, and 25 calories)

1 cup raw vegetables

½ cup cooked vegetables

Asparagus

Green beans

Beets

Broccoli

Brussels sprouts

Cabbage

Cauliflower

Eggplant

Greens (collard, mustard, turnip)

Kohlrabi

Leeks

Mushrooms

Okra

Onions

Peppers

Rutabaga

Spinach

Summer squash

Tomato

Turnips

Zucchini

FRUITS
(1 fruit exchange or 1 serving = 15 grams of carbohydrate, 0 protein, 0 fat, and 60 calories)

1 small apple (2" diameter)

½ cup unsweetened applesauce

3 medium apricots

1 small banana

¾ cup blackberries

¾ cup blueberries

⅓ cantaloupe (5" diameter)

1 cup cubed cantaloupe

12 cherries

1 ounce dried fruit

2 figs

½ grapefruit

15 grapes

⅛ honeydew (medium)

1 cup cubed honeydew

1 kiwi

½ mango

1 nectarine (2½" diameter)

1 orange (2½" diameter)

1 cup papaya

1 peach (2¾" diameter)

1 small pear

2 medium persimmons

¾ cup pineapple

2 plums (2" diameter)

3 prunes

2 tablespoons raisins

1 cup raspberries

1¼ cups strawberries

2 tangerines

1¼ cups watermelon

FAT-FREE OR LOW-FAT DAIRY
(1 fat-free milk exchange or 1 serving = 12 grams of carbohydrate, 8 grams of protein, 0 to 3 grams of fat, and 120 calories)

1 cup fat-free or low-fat (1%) milk

1 cup fat-free or low-fat buttermilk

1 cup low-fat soy milk, plain

½ cup evaporated skim milk

⅓ cup dry fat-free milk

¾ cup low-fat or fat-free yogurt, plain

(continued)

THE FOOD EXCHANGE GUIDE (*cont.*)

LEAN MEATS (3 OUNCES OF LEAN MEAT OR 1 SERVING = 3 MEAT EXCHANGES)
(1 lean meat exchange [unless otherwise specified] = 7 grams of protein, 0 to 3 grams of fat, and 35 to 55 calories)

1 ounce USDA select or choice grades of lean beef: round, sirloin, tenderloin, and flank steak

1 ounce lean pork

1 ounce skinless poultry

1 ounce fish

MEAT SUBSTITUTES
2 egg whites or ¼ cup egg substitute (counts as 1 lean meat exchange or 1 serving)

¼ cup cottage cheese (counts as 1 lean meat exchange or 1 serving)

1 ounce low-fat cheese (counts as 1 lean meat exchange or 1 serving)

½ cup cooked beans, peas, or legumes (counts as 1 lean meat exchange and 1 starch)

4 ounces or ½ cup tofu (counts as 1 lean meat exchange and 1 fat)

¼ cup tempeh (counts as 1 lean meat exchange and 1 fat)

ACCEPTABLE FATS
(1 fat exchange or 1 serving = 5 grams of fat and 45 calories)

⅛ avocado

1 teaspoon soft tub margarine (canola oil-based and trans fat–free)

1 teaspoon mayonnaise (canola oil-based)

1 tablespoon salad dressing (olive oil- or canola oil-based)

2 tablespoons reduced-fat salad dressing

1 teaspoon olive oil

1 teaspoon canola oil

1 teaspoon sesame oil

FREE FOODS
A free food is any food or drink that contains less than 20 calories or less than 5 grams of carbohydrate per serving. Foods with a serving size should be limited to three servings a day. (Be sure to spread them throughout the day.)

1 tablespoon fat-free cream cheese

Nonstick cooking spray

1 tablespoon fat-free sour cream

Coffee

Tea

Ketchup

Mustard

Lemon juice

Soy sauce (reduced sodium, use sparingly)

Seasonings

Fresh herbs

People with LDL Pattern A

People with LDL pattern A have a predominance of large, buoyant LDL (as opposed to people with LDL pattern B, who have a predominance of the atherogenic, small dense LDL). So LDL pattern A people are in comparatively good shape: The majority of their LDLs are the "not-so-bad" kind. Why do they need a special diet?

Well, you see something odd when you test some LDL pattern A people after they've been put on low-fat diets. Their LDL cholesterol goes down, but their apo B doesn't. What that tells us is that although the *amount* of LDL cholesterol has changed, the *number* of molecules of LDL hasn't. That means that on low-fat diets, some pattern A people actually change the way they carry their cholesterol: from the large, buoyant LDL particles to smaller, denser, more dangerous particles. Clearly, this is exactly the opposite of what we want to see! For this reason, patients with LDL pattern A belong on moderately low-fat diets, where fat makes up not less than 25 percent of the total calories.

A lot of you will greet this news with a sigh of relief. You're not unresponsive to diet after all! This piece of information does solve a lot of the mystery surrounding people's lack of success on the widely prescribed low-fat diet. For instance, women on low-fat diets often show less reduction in their LDL cholesterol than do men, and for years, this left cardiologists scratching their heads. But many premenopausal women are pattern A. There wasn't anything wrong with what they were doing: They simply required a more balanced diet with less severe restrictions on their intake of fats.

People with Multiple Metabolic Problems

Balance is the key to this diet, which is why it's the best possible option for people with certain combinations of these metabolic disorders.

At first glance, you could think that some of the dietary recommendations for these metabolic issues are contradictory. If the right thing to do for an apo E4 is a low-fat, high-carbohydrate diet, and the right thing to do for someone with high triglycerides is a lower-carbohydrate, higher-fat diet, then what are you supposed to do if you have both conditions at the same time!?!?

You go on this Diet Plan, which was developed with precisely this conundrum in mind.

Look at it this way: If you treat one condition at the expense of another, you're just going to end up a kind of perpetual seesaw, with your numbers bouncing from one side to the other. Treat the apo E4 problem, and you'll make the triglyceride problem worse; if you go after the triglycerides, you'll aggravate the apo E4 issue. Now, if you have a real red-alert score—an astronomically high triglyceride level of 2,000, say, your doctor might very well take this tack. He might want to focus exclusively on getting you out of the danger zone with those triglycerides, no matter what that diet did to your less-immediate apo E4 issue. But this is an extreme example. (If your triglycerides are 2,000, you'd better be under close physician supervision!) For most of you, the problem will be less radical, a little bit of both conditions. In that case, the most sensible plan is moderation.

THE WHOLE HEART DIET: DAILY EXCHANGES

- Nine servings of whole, unrefined grains, breads, cereals, and starchy vegetables.

- Six servings of vegetables. Include one high-vitamin-C source every day and one high-beta-carotene source every other day.

- Three servings of whole fruit, fresh or frozen.

- Three servings of fat-free or low-fat dairy. Substitute soy wherever possible.

- Six ounces of lean meat, fish, or skinless poultry. Use red meat three times or less a week. Incorporate fish at least twice during the week. Substitute soy products for meats wherever possible.

- One-half serving (½ ounce or 1 tablespoon) of nuts a day.

- Six servings of acceptable fats. Use only canola and olive oil; trans fat–free, canola-based margarines; and canola-based mayonnaise.

The truth is that these conditions don't really contradict each other. Apo E4s don't need to go on the kind of crazy, no-fat diet that's going to send their triglycerides soaring, and people with high triglycerides don't have to eliminate carbohydrates completely—they just have to make better choices about the kind of carbohydrates they eat. The Whole Heart Diet uses all of our nutritional building blocks to stabilize that seesaw so that you can dismount once and for all.

People Who Don't Yet Have a Complete Cardiac Fingerprint

It's helpful to know your metabolic issues before starting a Diet Plan. As we've seen, the wrong diet—even a supposedly healthy low-fat one, can be a real disaster unless you know what you're dealing with in advance. As you'll discover a little later, one of the strongest arguments against a severely low-fat diet is that people on very-low-fat diets tend to see a decrease in their HDL, or "good" cholesterol—the effect exactly opposite from the one that we'd like to see. People on severely low-fat diets also tend to show higher triglyceride levels. So the generic advice that people have been getting hasn't always helped their hearts, and in certain cases, it may even have hurt them.

If you haven't yet gotten your metabolic marker results, but are eager to start changing your eating habits immediately, you'll be perfectly safe starting with this diet. None of the Diet Plans in the Nutrition Prescription drop fat to the level where you're likely to see an increase in triglycerides and a decrease in HDL, but the Whole Heart Diet is designed to have a beneficial effect on your whole heart, no matter what your profile shows. For this reason, it's the plan we recommend to anyone looking generally to prevent coronary heart disease through diet.

DIET PLAN #1:
THE WHOLE HEART DIET

30% fat, 50% carbohydrates, 20% protein

THE WHOLE HEART DIET:
THE BUILDING BLOCK BREAKDOWN

Fat: 30% of calories

This is a moderately low-fat diet, which is good news for your heart and your taste buds!

Saturated: < 6% of calories

This translates to no more than 13 grams of saturated fat a day.

- Limit meat, poultry, and fish intake to 6 ounces a day. A 3-ounce serving is about the size of a deck of cards.

- Choose only very lean cuts of meats and limit red meat to three servings or less a week.

- Eat fish at least twice a week.

- Substitute soy products for meats wherever possible.

- Choose fat-free or low-fat dairy products instead of the full-fat alternatives.

Monounsaturated: Approximately 15% of calories

Limit added fats to 6 teaspoons a day. Added fats are the fats and oils that you add to foods, the oils that you use to sauté and make salad dressings, and the canola margarines you spread on bread. Substitute canola oil for margarine wherever possible.

- Use trans fat–free, canola-based, soft tub margarines.

- Use canola oil as your main cooking oil. It's a good source of monounsaturated fats and it also provides an omega-3 fatty acid. Use olive oil when cooking and in salad dressings (whenever the taste is preferred).

- Add ½ ounce (1 tablespoon) of nuts a day.

ONE-WEEK MENU PLANNING

The Whole Heart Diet

The following menu plans will give you 1 week of simple, easy-to-prepare meals that fit within the Whole Heart Diet. The nutrition advice and the suggested menu plans were developed by Lisa Sawrey-Kubicek, M.S., R.D., a nu-

Polyunsaturated: < 10% of calories

You'll get this amount easily from other foods in the diet. You don't have to add polyunsaturated oils to achieve this level.

<u>Carbohydrates:</u> 50% of calories

• Eat up to nine servings of unrefined, complex carbohydrates, like whole grain or multigrain bread, pasta, brown rice, and starchy vegetables a day. Limit refined carbohydrates.

• Eat at least six servings of vegetables a day.

• Cut sweets.

• Limit fruit to three servings a day.

<u>Protein:</u> 20% of calories

• Choose lower-fat sources of protein, like very lean meats, skinless poultry, fish, and egg whites.

• Eat fish at least twice a week.

• Try to have at least one meatless meal a week. Use protein-rich legumes such as lentils and beans instead of meat. Substitute soy products for meat wherever possible.

• Include three servings a day of fat-free or low-fat dairy products or low-fat, calcium-enriched soy milk.

■ *These recommendations are for a 2,000-calorie diet.*

tritionist who has worked with Dr. Superko since the inception of his program. Collaboration on the menus was provided by Kathy Hanuschak, R.D., L.D.N. These sample menus will get you started, and then you can use them as templates in combination with the Food Exchange Guide on page 164, to craft countless variations of your own.

DAY 1

Breakfast

½ pink grapefruit

½ cup cooked oatmeal

1 slice whole grain toast

1 teaspoon canola margarine

1 cup fat-free or low-fat (1%) milk

Coffee or tea with milk and sugar, if desired

Lunch

Salmon Sandwich

2 slices whole grain bread

3 ounces broiled salmon

½ cup lettuce and sliced tomato

2 teaspoons canola mayonnaise

Walnut Pear Salad

1 cup mixed salad greens

1 small sliced pear

1 tablespoon chopped walnuts

1 tablespoon vinaigrette (olive-oil based)

1 cup fat-free or low-fat (1%) milk

Snack

1 whole grain bagel

2 tablespoons fat-free cream cheese

Dinner

Dinner salad

3 ounces baked chicken breast

2 small red potatoes, halved, roasted with rosemary and 1 teaspoon olive oil

1 cup steamed green beans

½ cup steamed carrots

1 whole grain roll

½ cup fresh fruit salad

1 cup fat-free or low-fat (1%) milk

DAY 2

Breakfast

¾ cup bran flakes

2 tablespoons raisins

1 cup fat-free or low-fat (1%) milk

1 slice whole grain toast

1 teaspoon canola margarine

Coffee or tea with milk and sugar, if desired

Lunch

Chicken Soft Tacos

> Two 6-inch steamed corn tortillas
>
> 2 ounces cooked chicken, cut into thin strips
>
> 1 ounce shredded low-fat Monterey Jack cheese
>
> 1 cup lettuce and sliced tomato
>
> ½ cup salsa
>
> 2 tablespoons low-fat dressing

½ cup cubed mango

1 cup fat-free or low-fat (1%) milk

Snack

8 low-fat whole grain crackers

1 tablespoon almond butter

Dinner

> Dinner salad

3 ounces baked sole fillet

2 tablespoons fat-free sour cream

⅔ cup steamed brown rice

1 teaspoon canola oil or canola margarine

1 cup steamed broccoli

½ cup blueberries

1 cup fat-free or low-fat (1%) milk

DAY 3

Breakfast

¾ cup shredded wheat cereal

1 cup fat-free or low-fat (1%) milk

½ cup sliced strawberries

> Coffee or tea with milk and sugar, if desired

Lunch

Turkey Sandwich

> 2 slices rye bread
>
> 3 ounces roast turkey
>
> ½ cup lettuce and sliced tomato
>
> 2 teaspoons canola mayonnaise
>
> 1 teaspoon Dijon mustard

Spring Salad

> 1 cup mixed salad greens
>
> ½ cup grated carrot and cucumber
>
> 1 tablespoon citrus vinaigrette (olive-oil based)

1 small peach

1 cup fat-free or low-fat (1%) milk

Snack

2 slices whole grain bread

1 tablespoon natural peanut butter

Dinner

> Dinner salad

3 ounces broiled lean sirloin beef steak with 1 cup mushrooms sautéed in 1 teaspoon olive oil

1 medium baked potato

2 tablespoons fat-free sour cream

½ cup steamed carrots

½ cup steamed broccoli

1 teaspoon canola oil or canola margarine

1 whole grain roll

1 small baked apple with cinnamon

1 cup fat-free or low-fat (1%) milk

DAY 4

Breakfast

Egg Sandwich

Sauté:

½ cup egg whites or egg substitute in 1 teaspoon canola oil or canola margarine

2 slices whole grain toast

1 teaspoon canola margarine

2 tangerines

1 cup fat-free or low-fat (1%) milk

Coffee or tea with milk and sugar, if desired

Lunch

1 cup vegetarian lentil soup

1 whole grain roll

Italian Salad

1 cup mixed Italian greens

½ cup grated carrot, green onion, chopped tomato

1 tablespoon balsamic vinaigrette (olive-oil based)

1 apple

1 cup fat-free or low-fat (1%) milk

Snack

8 low-fat whole grain crackers

1 tablespoon almond butter

Dinner

Dinner salad

3 ounces sea bass

1 teaspoon canola margarine

½ cup low-sodium crushed tomatoes

1 cup steamed brown rice

½ cup steamed collard greens

1 poached pear

1 cup fat-free or low-fat (1%) milk

DAY 5

Breakfast

Garden Omelet

Sauté:

½ cup diced vegetables

½ cup egg whites or egg substitute in 1 teaspoon canola oil or canola margarine

2 slices whole grain toast

1 teaspoon canola margarine

1 cup fat-free or low-fat (1%) milk

1 small orange

Coffee or tea with milk and sugar, if desired

Lunch

Chicken Sandwich

 2 slices rye bread

 3 ounces baked chicken

 ½ cup lettuce and sliced tomato

 2 teaspoons canola mayonnaise

 1 teaspoon Dijon mustard

½ cup raw baby carrots

1 cup seedless grapes

1 cup fat-free or low-fat (1%) milk

Snack

½ whole grain bagel

1 tablespoon almond butter

DAY 6

Breakfast

¾ cup bran flakes

½ cup sliced strawberries

1 cup fat-free or low-fat (1%) milk

 Coffee or tea with milk and sugar, if desired

Dinner

Dinner salad

Pasta Primavera

1½ cups cooked whole wheat rotini

 1 cup marinara sauce with garlic and herbs

 1½ cups assorted vegetables sautéed in 1 teaspoon olive oil

 1 ounce shredded low-fat mozzarella cheese

 1 tablespoon chopped fresh basil

1 whole grain roll

1 small sliced peach

1 cup fat-free or low-fat (1%) milk

Lunch

Grilled Soy Burger

 1 whole grain bun

 1 grilled soy burger

 1 ounce low-fat Cheddar cheese

 ½ cup lettuce and sliced tomato

 2 teaspoons canola mayonnaise

 2 teaspoons ketchup

 1 teaspoon Dijon mustard

½ cup steamed carrots

1 teaspoon canola oil or canola margarine

Spring Salad

 1 cup mixed salad greens

 ½ cup grated carrot and cucumber

 1 tablespoon citrus vinaigrette (olive-oil based)

1 cup cubed cantaloupe

1 cup fat-free or low-fat (1%) milk

Snack

- 1 multigrain English muffin
- 1 tablespoon natural peanut butter

Dinner

Dinner salad

- 3 ounces turkey cutlet
- ½ cup baked sweet potato
- 1 teaspoon canola margarine
- ⅔ cup steamed brown rice
- 1 cup steamed green beans
- 2 tablespoons unsweetened cranberry sauce
- 1 cup fat-free or low-fat (1%) milk

DAY 7

Breakfast

- ¾ cup multigrain cereal
- 1 cup low-fat soy milk, enriched with calcium
- 1 small sliced peach

Coffee or tea with milk and sugar, if desired

Lunch

Chili with Cornbread

- 1 bowl low-fat vegetarian black bean chili topped with
- 1 ounce shredded low-fat Monterey Jack cheese
- ½ cup salsa
- 2 tablespoons fat-free sour cream
- 1 tablespoon green onion

One 2-inch piece cornbread

Spring Salad

- 1 cup mixed salad greens
- ½ cup grated carrot and cucumber
- 1 tablespoon vinaigrette (olive-oil based)
- 1 tablespoon slivered almonds
- 1 cup fat-free or low-fat (1%) milk

Snack

- 3 cups air-popped popcorn, plain
- 1 small pear

Dinner

Dinner salad

- 3 ounces roast pork tenderloin
- 1 cup baked sweet potato
- 1 teaspoon canola margarine
- 1 cup steamed turnip greens
- ½ cup steamed turnips
- ½ cup blueberries
- 1 cup fat-free or low-fat (1%) milk

DIET PLAN #2
THE MORE-FAT, LOW-FAT DIET

You read it right! We're adding *more* fat to your low-fat diet.

If you're already following a low-fat diet for your heart, you're going to be pretty pleased to see how comparatively liberal this "lower-fat" Diet Plan is. And you'll be pleased by the results you get as well! This Diet Plan is lower in fat than the others in the Nutrition Prescription, and it's very low in *saturated fat*. But it's nowhere near as prohibitive as many of the low-fat diets out there. So why am I *adding* fat to your low-fat diet?

- Diets too severely restrictive in fat can actually lower your HDL—the good cholesterol with all the protective benefits to your heart.
- Most low-fat diets don't differentiate between unhealthy, artery-clogging saturated fats and more heart-healthy unsaturated fats. We do!
- Most low-fat diets don't differentiate between "junk" carbohydrates (the simple, refined, sugary ones) and "quality" carbohydrates (complex, slow-burning ones that are low on the glycemic index). We'll teach you the difference.

How low fat is *too low fat?*

There are a few scientific reasons for a more lenient approach to fat.

First of all, people on severely low-fat diets often experience a reduction in beneficial, protective HDL cholesterol. This is the wrong direction to be going in, and in my opinion, it's madness to adopt a diet plan that's going to rob your heart of protection.

Moreover, these extremely low-fat diets don't seem to confer any extra benefit in LDL-cholesterol reduction. Yes, LDL does go down on a low-fat diet, and that's unquestionably a desired outcome. So does it go down even more on a super-low-fat diet? Apparently not. There doesn't seem to be any added advantage to dropping fat below 25 percent. So you're cheating your body out of an ingredient it needs—and your taste buds out of an ingredient they want—and you won't even see an appreciable difference in your blood work.

A NOTE ON HOMOCYSTEINE AND YOUR DIET

Homocysteine is formed in the blood after the body metabolizes methionine, an essential amino acid. Usually, the homocysteine is also metabolized and removed from your body as a matter of course, unless you're someone who's inherited an inability to do this efficiently, which means that high levels of homocysteine remain in the blood. Elevated levels of homocysteine have been linked to coronary heart disease, and lowering homocysteine levels has been linked to less heart artery blockage following the cardiac procedure called angioplasty.

You don't eat homocysteine, so you can't avoid it in food. But you can use diet to address this high-homocysteine issue.

First and foremost, you need to increase your intake of foods rich in vitamins B_6, B_{12}, and folate, like beans, broccoli, and spinach. (These vitamins will be covered in great detail in the supplement section.)

Restrict your level of methionine. Methionine levels are high in meat, poultry, fish, and dairy products. In a small pilot study, men who consumed a low-methionine diet normalized their homocysteine values in just 3 weeks. One study doesn't make protocol, but it makes sense that limiting methionine will reduce your levels of homocysteine. The terrific results in this study may also have been a result of increased folate consumption; the low-methionine diet was necessarily high in fruits and vegetables.

Fats Aren't All Created Equal

Many low-fat diets fail to differentiate between the different kinds of fat, which is ridiculous! As we know, saturated fat is the type of fat that has the greatest effect on lipid levels, so that's the one I want you to avoid.

Saturated fat is kept low in all the Diet Plans, but it's especially important to limit it in this diet, since we know you're super-sensitive to fat. When you eat fat on this Diet Plan (and you will be able to), it should be one of the monounsaturated ones.

THE MORE-FAT, LOW-FAT DIET: DAILY EXCHANGES

- Up to 11 servings of whole, unrefined grains, breads, cereals, and starchy vegetables.

- Six servings of vegetables. Include one high-vitamin-C source every day and one high-beta-carotene source every other day.

- Three servings of whole fruit, fresh or frozen.

- Three servings of fat-free or low-fat dairy. Substitute soy wherever possible.

- Five ounces of lean meat, fish, or skinless poultry. Use red meat three times or less a week. Incorporate fish at least twice during the week. Substitute soy products for meats wherever possible.

- Five and a half servings of acceptable fats. Use only canola and olive oil; trans fat–free, canola-based margarines; and canola-based mayonnaise.

Carbs Aren't All Created Equal Either

Another difference between this Diet Plan and some other low-fat diets is a pronounced focus on quality carbohydrates. People on cardiac-care diets tend to concentrate pretty exclusively on fat. They don't care what kind of carbs they're eating, just as long as those foods are low in fat.

And so the destructive cycle begins: Their diets end up having too many refined carbohydrates high on the glycemic index, and that increases their blood sugars. Not surprisingly, compliance with these diets is often accompanied by an increase in triglycerides and weight gain.

Not exactly the desired effect! The focus of this Diet Plan is on lowering fat, but that doesn't mean you can compensate by eating all the sugar you want. If you're going to go on a Diet Plan to improve your lipid levels, it should actually improve your lipid levels—not make some of them better at the expense of the others.

Since we know that both fructose (the sugar found in fruit) and sucrose (table sugar) increase triglyceride levels, we keep those two sugars at a minimum in this diet. And I will continue to encourage you to watch the *type* of carbohydrates that you eat in the place of some of these fats. We'll show you how to choose "quality" carbohydrates over "junk" by choosing fruits over sweets and whole grains over refined foods as often as possible.

Note: Your triglycerides should always be monitored when you're adopting a new way of eating. Increased triglycerides could be an indication of the expression of the LDL pattern B trait—or a sign that the pattern B trait is getting worse, and that's something you're going to want to treat immediately.

If your triglycerides do increase, take these measures to lower them.

- Eliminate alcohol.
- Eliminate sweets. Limit fruit to two servings a day.
- Watch out for refined carbohydrates (white flour, white rice, starchy vegetables) or other hidden sugars in your diet—and eliminate them.
- Make sure you're getting enough exercise, which will burn excess triglycerides away.
- Consider losing weight, if applicable. Triglycerides are often high in people who are overweight. Losing even as little as 10 pounds can dramatically improve your lipid levels.

If following these guidelines doesn't help reduce your elevated triglycerides, then you should talk to your doctor about a diet that restricts carbohydrates, such as the Better-Carbohydrate, Lower-Carbohydrate Diet in this Nutrition Prescription.

Who Should Use This Diet Plan?

- People with LDL pattern B
- People with high apo B
- People with apo E4

People with LDL pattern B

People with LDL pattern B have a predominance of small, dense LDL particles—an intensely atherogenic form of the LDL particle.

You may remember the pattern B paradox: Coronary heart disease progresses much more rapidly in people with LDL pattern B, but these people also respond very well to treatment. And one of the treatment paths that people with LDL pattern B respond especially strongly to is diet! An individual with LDL pattern B on a low-fat diet shows *twice* the reduction in LDL-C as an individual with LDL pattern A. The news gets even better: on a low-fat diet, pattern Bs show reductions in the number of those small dense LDL particles. That means that, with the right diet alone, you can actually begin to convert yourself from the atherogenic, dangerous LDL pattern B to a much less dangerous LDL pattern A!

People with high apo B

There's one apo B, and only one, on every LDL particle. So if your apo B is high, we know that you have a high number of circulating LDL particles, and that's dangerous. As we know, a low-fat diet is one of the best ways to reduce that number.

Soy proteins have also been shown to decrease the level of circulating apo B, so if you have a problem with apo B, I'd advise you to replace as many animal proteins (dairy and meat) in this Diet Plan as you can with soy proteins.

People with apo E4

Apo E4 people are like LDL pattern B people: They're at higher risk of disease, but they're also super-respondent to treatment, notably a low-fat diet. People with this apo E4 allele, or gene type, respond very well to a low-fat diet, with bigger reductions in their LDL cholesterol than people with either the apo E3 (more common) or apo E2 (less common) allele.

DIET PLAN #2:
THE MORE-FAT, LOW-FAT DIET

25% fat, 55% carbohydrates, 20% protein

A low-fat diet works for apo E4s because they tend to keep fat in circulation longer; the lipoproteins with E4s attached are more attractive to those LDL receptors in the liver that suck LDL cholesterol and some other lipoproteins out of the bloodstream. This results in more cholesterol inside the liver cell. When the liver doesn't feel that it "needs" cholesterol, it decreases the

THE MORE-FAT, LOW-FAT DIET:
THE BUILDING BLOCK BREAKDOWN

Fat: 25% of calories

Saturated: < 6% of calories

This translates to no more than 13 grams of saturated fat a day.

- Limit meat, poultry, and fish intake to 5 ounces a day. A 3-ounce serving is about the size of a deck of cards. You can have a 2-ounce serving at lunch and a 3-ounce serving at dinner.

- Choose only very lean cuts of meats and limit red meat to three servings or less a week.

- Eat fish at least twice a week.

- Substitute soy products for meats wherever possible.

- Choose fat-free or low-fat dairy products instead of the full-fat alternatives.

Monounsaturated: Approximately 10% of calories

Limit added fats to 5.5 teaspoons a day. Added fats are the fats and oils that you add to foods, the oils that you use to sauté and make salad dressings, and the canola margarines you spread on bread. Substitute canola oil for margarine wherever possible.

- Use trans fat–free, canola-based, soft tub margarines.

- Use canola oil as your main cooking oil. It's a good source of monounsaturated fats and it also provides an omega-3 fatty acid. Use olive oil when cooking and in salad dressings (whenever the taste is preferred).

number of receptors it's got pulling cholesterol out of the blood, which means that there's more of it out there—and you have higher blood LDL-C values. Apo E4 is one of the most common causes for high levels of LDL cholesterol. So low fat is a good thing for you, but it's not a "how low can you go" situation. It's the same story with the apo E4s as it is with the pattern Bs: Low fat

Polyunsaturated: < 10% of calories
You'll get this amount easily from other foods in the diet. You don't have to add polyunsaturated oils to achieve this level.

Carbohydrates: 55% of calories

• Eat up to 11 servings of unrefined, complex carbohydrates, like whole grain or multigrain bread, pasta, brown rice, and starchy vegetables a day. Limit refined carbohydrates.

• Eat at least six servings of vegetables a day.

• Limit fruit to three servings a day.

• Avoid fruit juice.

• Strictly limit other sources of sugar.

Protein: 20% of calories

• Choose lower-fat sources of protein, like very lean meats, skinless poultry, fish, and egg whites.

• Eat fish at least twice a week.

• Try to have at least one meatless meal a week. Use protein-rich legumes such as lentils and beans instead of meat. Substitute soy products for meat wherever possible.

• Include three servings a day of fat-free or low-fat dairy products or low-fat, calcium-enriched soy milk.

■ *These recommendations are for a 2,000-calorie diet.*

is really good, but super-low fat doesn't seem to be any better. Studies have shown that there is little further benefit in LDL cholesterol reduction when fat intake goes below 25 percent.

A Note about Alcohol

I don't recommend alcohol for anyone pursuing a heart-healthy diet, but it's especially important to cut it out if you're having a problem with any of the blood-sugar issues, including elevated insulin levels and triglycerides.

Alcoholic beverages (beer, wine, hard liquor) are common contributors to elevated triglyceride levels. For some individuals, even a moderate intake of alcohol (such as four or five glasses of wine a week) is enough to significantly raise triglyceride levels. You can find out if your triglycerides are super-sensitive to alcohol by cutting it out for a week and then having your blood tested.

Since triglycerides tend to go up when you're on a lower-fat diet, you might want to consider cutting back on the alcohol you consume. In fact, if you're having a hard time keeping your triglycerides under 200 milligrams per deciliter, you'll want to severely limit your alcohol intake (or even better, cut it out entirely).

ONE-WEEK MENU PLANNING

The More-Fat, Low-Fat Diet

The following menu plans will give you 1 week of simple, easy-to-prepare meals that fit within the More-Fat, Low-Fat Diet. The nutrition advice and the suggested menu plans were developed by Lisa Sawrey-Kubicek, M.S., R.D., a nutritionist who has worked with Dr. Superko since the inception of his program. Collaboration on the menus was provided by Kathy Hanuschak, R.D., L.D.N. These sample menus will get you started, and then you can use them as templates in combination with the Food Exchange Guide on page 164 to craft countless variations of your own.

DAY 1

Breakfast

1 cup cubed honeydew

¾ cup shredded wheat cereal

1 cup fat-free or low-fat (1%) milk

1 whole grain bagel

2 tablespoons fat-free cream cheese

Coffee or tea with milk and sugar, if desired

Lunch

Chicken in Pita

1 whole wheat pita

2 ounces cooked chicken breast

½ cup lettuce and sliced tomato

2 teaspoons canola mayonnaise

Mixed Greens and Fruit Salad

1 cup mixed salad greens

1 small sliced pear

1 tablespoon balsamic vinaigrette (olive-oil based)

1 cup fat-free or low-fat (1%) milk

Snack

8 low-fat whole grain crackers

½ cup salsa

Dinner

Dinner salad

Linguine with Red Clam Sauce

1½ cups cooked linguine

½ cup marinara sauce with garlic and herbs

3 ounces chopped clams

1 small multigrain roll

1 teaspoon canola margarine

½ cup steamed vegetable medley

½ teaspoon canola oil or canola margarine

½ cup fresh fruit salad

1 cup fat-free or low-fat (1%) milk

DAY 2

Breakfast

1 cup cooked oatmeal

½ cup stewed apples

1 whole grain English muffin

1 teaspoon canola margarine

1 cup fat-free or low-fat (1%) milk

Coffee or tea with milk and sugar, if desired

Lunch

Grilled Soy Burger

1 whole grain bun

1 grilled soy burger

½ cup lettuce and sliced tomato

2 teaspoons canola mayonnaise

2 teaspoons ketchup

1 teaspoon Dijon mustard

1 cup steamed cauliflower and broccoli

1 cup fat-free or low-fat (1%) milk

Snack

8 low-fat whole grain crackers

1 small orange

DAY 3

Breakfast

¾ cup bran flakes

2 tablespoons raisins

1 cup fat-free or low-fat (1%) milk

1 whole grain bagel

1 teaspoon canola margarine

Coffee or tea with milk and sugar, if desired

Lunch

Turkey Sandwich

2 slices whole grain bread

2 ounces roast turkey breast

½ cup lettuce and sliced tomato

2 teaspoons canola mayonnaise

1 cup tomato soup

1 cup fat-free or low-fat (1%) milk

Dinner

Dinner salad

3 ounces grilled chicken breast

2 tablespoons low-sodium barbecue sauce

½ cup steamed peas and carrots

½ cup steamed butternut squash

½ cup cooked orzo

½ teaspoon canola oil or canola margarine

1 slice whole grain bread

1 teaspoon canola margarine

¾ cup pineapple chunks

1 cup fat-free or low-fat plain yogurt

Snack

8 low-fat crackers

1 small apple

Dinner

Dinner salad

Spaghetti with Turkey

1½ cups cooked spaghetti

1 cup marinara sauce with garlic and herbs

3 ounces 99% fat-free ground turkey

1 cup steamed broccoli

1 teaspoon canola oil or canola margarine

1 cup cubed papaya

1 cup fat-free or low-fat (1%) milk

DAY 4

Breakfast

½ pink grapefruit

1 cup cooked oatmeal

1 whole grain bagel

2 tablespoons fat-free cream cheese

1 cup fat-free or low-fat (1%) milk

Coffee or tea with milk and sugar, if desired

Lunch

Chicken-Avocado Salad

  1 cup mixed salad greens with spinach

  2 ounces cooked chicken

  ⅛ avocado, peeled and sliced

  2 tablespoons low-fat dressing

1 pumpernickel roll

1 teaspoon canola margarine

1 cup fat-free or low-fat (1%) milk

Snack

8 low-fat whole grain crackers

1 small pear

Dinner

Dinner salad

3 ounces broiled lean sirloin beef steak with 1 cup mushrooms sautéed in 1 teaspoon olive oil

1 small baked potato

2 tablespoons fat-free sour cream

1 cup sliced red beets

1 whole wheat roll

½ teaspoon canola margarine

½ cup fresh fruit salad

1 cup fat-free or low-fat (1%) milk

DAY 5

Breakfast

Two 4-inch buckwheat pancakes

½ cup sliced strawberries

2 tablespoons fat-free or low-fat plain yogurt

¾ cup fat-free or low-fat (1%) milk

Coffee or tea with milk and sugar, if desired

Lunch

- 1 cup low-fat vegetarian black bean chili topped with
- 2 tablespoons fat-free sour cream
- 2 tablespoons salsa
- 2 tablespoons chopped green onion

Spinach Salad

- 1 cup baby spinach
- ½ cup mandarin oranges
- 1 tablespoon citrus vinaigrette (olive-oil based)
- 1 multigrain roll
- 1 cup fat-free or low-fat (1%) milk

Snack

- 1 whole wheat English muffin
- ½ cup salsa

Dinner

- Dinner salad
- 3 ounces grilled salmon steak
- ⅔ cup steamed brown rice
- ½ teaspoon canola oil or canola margarine
- 1 cup steamed broccoli and cauliflower
- 1 whole grain roll
- 1 teaspoon canola margarine
- 1 cup cubed cantaloupe
- 1 cup fat-free or low-fat (1%) milk

DAY 6

Breakfast

- ¾ cup multigrain cereal
- 1 cup fat-free or low-fat (1%) milk
- 1 small sliced peach
- 2 slices whole grain toast
- 2 teaspoons canola margarine
- Coffee or tea with milk and sugar, if desired

Lunch

Chicken and Pasta with Marinara

- ½ cup cooked angel hair pasta
- 1 cup marinara sauce with garlic and herbs
- 2 ounces cooked chicken breast
- ½ cup steamed green beans
- 1 teaspoon canola oil or canola margarine
- 1 cup cubed cantaloupe
- 1 cup fat-free or low-fat (1%) milk

Snack

- 3 cups air-popped popcorn
- 2 tangerines

Dinner

Dinner salad

3 ounces baked haddock with fresh lemon juice

1 cup steamed brown rice

1 teaspoon canola oil or canola margarine

DAY 7

Breakfast

¾ cup shredded wheat cereal

1 cup fat-free or low-fat (1%) milk

½ cup sliced strawberries

1 whole grain bagel

2 tablespoons fat-free cream cheese

Coffee or tea with milk and sugar, if desired

Lunch

Black Bean Burrito

1 8-inch whole wheat tortilla

½ cup cooked black beans

⅓ cup steamed brown rice

1 ounce shredded low-fat Monterey Jack cheese

½ cup salsa

1 ear corn on the cob

1 teaspoon canola margarine

Salad

1 cup mixed greens

½ cup lettuce and sliced cucumber

1 tablespoon vinaigrette (olive-oil based)

1 cup fat-free or low-fat (1%) milk

½ cup stewed zucchini and tomatoes

½ cup steamed carrots

½ teaspoon canola oil or canola margarine

1 cup fat-free or low-fat (1%) milk

Snack

1 cup vegetable soup

4 low-fat whole grain crackers

1 apple

Dinner

Dinner salad

3 ounces top-round London broil

1 small baked potato

1 teaspoon canola margarine

1 cup steamed vegetable medley

½ teaspoon canola oil or canola margarine

1 slice whole grain bread

1 teaspoon canola margarine

3 apricots

1 cup fat-free or low-fat (1%) milk

DIET PLAN #3
THE BETTER-CARBOHYDRATE, LOWER-CARBOHYDRATE DIET

This Diet Plan is lower in carbohydrates than the other plans in the Nutrition Prescription. You're probably thinking: "But isn't a low-fat, high-carbohydrate diet the standard recommendation for cardiac health?" Yes, a low-fat diet is a standard recommendation. And for many people, it's a mistake.

- Low-fat diets can make blood-sugar levels soar. Considering the link between diabetes and coronary heart disease, we can't afford to stand by while your blood-sugar levels climb unchecked.
- Unlike other low-carb diets, this isn't one of those all bacon-eggs-cheese-and-red-meat extravaganzas—I believe those diets put your heart at risk!

This isn't a no-carbohydrate diet, just a lower-carbohydrate diet, because we're going to be paying close attention to the *kind* and *quality* of carbs you eat, as well as the amount of them.

Diabetes and Coronary Heart Disease

A low-fat diet that relies heavily on refined carbohydrates can make blood-sugar levels soar. Diabetes and insulin resistance are shocking risk factors for coronary heart disease, and almost all diabetics die of coronary heart disease. When we consider how closely diabetes and prediabetic conditions are linked to coronary heart disease, it becomes very clear that we can't treat your heart by standing by while your blood sugar skyrockets.

This is one of the most devastating underlying metabolic factors, and we have to address it. Luckily, it's another one of the conditions that reacts robustly to dietary measures. The Better-Carbohydrate, Lower-Carbohydrate Diet is designed to tackle the issue of sugars in the blood, without driving you to the opposite, carbohydrate-free extreme.

THE BETTER-CARBOHYDRATE, LOWER-CARBOHYDRATE DIET: DAILY EXCHANGES

- Up to seven servings of whole, unrefined grains, breads, cereals, and starchy vegetables

- At least six servings of vegetables. Include one high-vitamin-C source every day and one high-beta-carotene source every other day.

- Up to three servings of whole fruit, fresh or frozen. No fruit juice.

- Include three servings of fat-free or low-fat dairy. Substitute soy wherever possible.

- Six ounces lean meat, fish, or skinless poultry. Use red meat three times or less a week. Incorporate fish at least twice during the week. Substitute soy products for meats wherever possible.

- One serving (1 ounce or 2 tablespoons) of nuts a day.

- Seven servings of acceptable fats. Use only canola and olive oil; trans fat–free, canola-based margarines; and canola-based mayonnaise.

Pass the saturated fat?

You will notice some differences between this Diet Plan and the other "low-carb" diets you've read or heard about. First of all, although this Diet Plan does allow for more fat than the other diets in the Nutrition Prescription, we're not subscribing to the "eat-all-the-fat-you-want" doctrine that is espoused in some of today's most popular low-carb diets. I do not condone diets that encourage you to sit down to a breakfast featuring bacon and eggs, followed by a steak topped off with a wheel of Brie. As far as I'm concerned, those diets aren't only poor science, they're completely counterintuitive. We know without a doubt that saturated fat is bad for your heart. How could any diet that allows unlimited consumption of it possibly be good for you?

The Better-Carbohydrate, Lower-Carbohydrate Diet is designed to keep cardiotoxic saturated-fat consumption low by substituting some of the carbohydrates with monounsaturated oils. So you do get to eat a relatively liberal amount of good-tasting fats. But hold that burger—you still have to concentrate on keeping saturated-fat levels down.

Make Your Carbs Count

Since we know that you're sensitive to carbohydrates, it's doubly important that the carbs you do eat are the right ones. I don't merely want to reduce the amount of carbohydrates you eat; I want to change the *kind* of carbohydrates you consume.

Numerous studies have shown that high-carbohydrate diets cause increases in triglycerides and decreases in HDL-C. This response has been shown to be influenced by the amount as well as the *type* of carbohydrate consumed. Simple carbohydrates such as sucrose (table sugar) have been linked to an increased production of triglycerides. And high-glycemic foods such as refined white bread can increase circulating insulin levels.

When you choose foods low on the glycemic index—that means whole grains and no refined flours, with limited starchy vegetables and very limited sweets—you get the best of both worlds. On this Diet Plan, you get all the benefits (and the taste!) of carbohydrates, without the elevated blood sugar—or the corresponding elevation in coronary heart disease risk.

Who Should Use This Diet Plan?

- People with elevated insulin
- People with high triglycerides

People with Elevated Insulin

People with high insulin levels need to control the amount of sugar circulating in their bloodstream, and since a higher-carbohydrate diet increases blood sugars, one way to reduce insulin is by cutting the amount of carbohydrates you consume. Reducing refined carbohydrates is also essential. The Better-Carbohydrate, Lower-Carbohydrate Diet will show you how to do both of those things by replacing excess carbohydrates with protein and "good fats," and those refined carbohydrates with slow-releasing, blood-sugar-leveling whole grains. Once again, think of your ancestors. Is your body designed to eat refined sugar, or complex carbohydrates in the form of whole grains?

People with High Triglycerides

High triglycerides are intrinsically linked to high levels of blood sugar, and high levels of triglycerides are a strong independent risk factor for heart attack.

Reducing your carbohydrate intake—especially "junk" carbs like simple sugars and processed starches—and limiting alcohol can make an enormous difference, and that's where we start with this diet. And don't ignore weight loss!

A Note about Alcohol

Again, I don't recommend alcohol for anyone pursuing a heart-healthy diet, but it's especially important to cut it out if you're having a problem with any of the blood-sugar issues, like insulin and triglycerides.

Alcoholic beverages (beer, wine, hard liquor) are common contributors to elevated triglyceride levels. For some individuals, even a moderate intake of alcohol (such as four or five glasses of wine a week) is enough to significantly raise triglyceride levels. You can find out if your triglycerides are super-sensitive to alcohol by cutting it out for a week and then having your blood tested.

If you're having a hard time keeping your triglycerides under 200 milligrams per deciliter, you'll want to severely limit your alcohol intake (or even better, cut it out entirely).

DIET PLAN #3: THE BETTER-CARBOHYDRATE, LOWER-CARBOHYDRATE DIET

35% fat, 45% carbohydrates, 20% protein

THE BETTER-CARBOHYDRATE, LOWER-CARBOHYDRATE DIET: THE BUILDING BLOCK BREAKDOWN

<u>Fat:</u> 35% of calories

Saturated: < 6% of calories

This translates to no more than 13 grams of saturated fat a day.

- Limit meat, poultry, and fish intake to 6 ounces a day. A 3-ounce serving is about the size of a deck of cards.

- Choose only very lean cuts of meats and limit red meat to three servings or less a week.

- Eat fish at least twice a week.

- Substitute soy products for meats wherever possible.

- Choose fat-free or low-fat dairy products instead of the full-fat alternatives.

Monounsaturated: Approximately 20% of calories

Limit added fats to 7 teaspoons a day. Added fats are the fats and oils that you add to foods, the oils that you use to sauté and make salad dressings, and the canola margarines you spread on bread. Substitute canola oil for margarine wherever possible.

- Use trans fat–free, canola-based, soft tub margarines.

- Use canola oil as your main cooking oil. It's a good source of monounsaturated fats and it also provides an omega-3 fatty acid. Use olive oil when cooking and in salad dressings (whenever the taste is preferred).

- Add 1 ounce (2 tablespoons) of nuts a day.

ONE-WEEK MENU PLANNING

The Better-Carbohydrate, Lower-Carbohydrate Diet

The following menu plans will give you 1 week of simple, easy-to-prepare meals that fit within the Better-Carbohydrate, Lower-Carbohydrate Diet. The nutrition advice and the suggested menu plans were developed by Lisa

Polyunsaturated: < 10% of calories

You'll get this amount easily from other foods in the diet. You don't have to add polyunsaturated oils to achieve this level.

<u>Carbohydrates:</u> 45% of calories

• Eat up to seven servings of unrefined, complex carbohydrates, like whole grain or multigrain bread, pasta, brown rice, and starchy vegetables a day. Limit refined carbohydrates.

• Eat at least six servings of vegetables a day.

• Limit fruits to three servings a day.

• No other source of sugar is allowed.

<u>Protein:</u> 20% of calories

• Choose lower-fat sources of protein, like lean meats, skinless poultry, fish, and egg whites.

• Eat fish at least twice a week.

• Try to have at least one meatless meal a week. Use protein-rich legumes such as lentils and beans instead of meat. Substitute soy products for meat wherever possible.

• Include three servings of fat-free or low-fat dairy products or low-fat, calcium-enriched soy milk.

■ *These recommendations are for a 2,000-calorie diet.*

Sawrey-Kubicek, M.S., R.D., a nutritionist who has worked with Dr. Superko since the inception of his program. Collaboration on menus was provided by Kathy Hanuschak, R.D., L.D.N. These sample menus will get you started, and then you can use them as templates in combination with the Food Exchange Guide on page 164 to craft countless variations of your own.

DAY 1

Breakfast

Egg Scramble

Sauté:

½ cup egg whites or egg substitute in 1 teaspoon canola oil or canola margarine

1 whole grain bagel

½ cup fresh fruit salad

1 cup fat-free or low-fat (1%) milk

Coffee or tea with milk and sugar, if desired

Lunch

Hummus Sandwich

1 whole wheat pita

⅓ cup hummus

½ cup lettuce and sliced tomato

½ cup sliced cucumber and sprouts

1 tablespoon vinaigrette (olive-oil based)

1 cup steamed broccoli and cauliflower

1 teaspoon canola oil or canola margarine

1 cup fat-free or low-fat (1%) milk

Snack

1 small apple

2 tablespoons almond butter

Dinner

Dinner salad

3 ounces roast pork tenderloin

½ cup baked sweet potato

1 teaspoon canola margarine

1 cup steamed Brussels sprouts

1 teaspoon canola oil or canola margarine

½ cup sliced red beets

1 slice whole grain bread

½ cup unsweetened applesauce

1 cup fat-free or low-fat (1%) milk

DAY 2

Breakfast

½ pink grapefruit

½ cup cooked oatmeal

1 multigrain bagel

1 teaspoon canola margarine

1 cup fat-free or low-fat (1%) milk

Coffee or tea with milk and sugar, if desired

Lunch

Chicken Sandwich

3 ounces baked chicken breast

2 slices whole grain bread

½ cup lettuce and sliced tomato

2 teaspoons canola mayonnaise

Spinach Salad

1 cup baby spinach

¼ cup raspberries

1 tablespoon raspberry vinaigrette (olive-oil based)

Snack

1 cup fat-free or low-fat plain yogurt

½ small banana

1 tablespoon chopped walnuts

Dinner

Dinner salad

3 ounces grilled chicken breast

2 tablespoons low-sodium barbecue sauce

1 cup cooked orzo with 1 tablespoon slivered almonds

1 teaspoon canola oil or canola margarine

1½ cups steamed vegetable medley

1 teaspoon canola oil or canola margarine

½ cup fresh fruit salad

1 cup fat-free or low-fat (1%) milk

DAY 3

Breakfast

¾ cup shredded wheat cereal

1 cup fat-free or low-fat (1%) milk

1 small sliced peach

Coffee or tea with milk and sugar, if desired

Lunch

Grilled Soy Burger

1 whole grain bun

1 grilled soy burger

1 ounce low-fat Cheddar cheese

½ cup lettuce and sliced tomato

2 teaspoons canola mayonnaise

2 teaspoons ketchup

1 teaspoon Dijon mustard

Spring Salad

½ cup mixed salad greens

½ cup grated carrot and cucumber

1 tablespoon sunflower seeds

1 tablespoon balsamic vinaigrette (olive-oil based)

1 small banana

1 cup fat-free or low-fat (1%) milk

Snack

4 low-fat whole grain crackers

1 tablespoon natural peanut butter

½ cup seedless grapes

Dinner

Dinner salad

3 ounces grilled chicken breast

1 small red potato, halved, roasted with rosemary and 1 teaspoon olive oil

½ cup steamed broccoli

½ cup steamed carrots

1 teaspoon canola oil or canola margarine

1 whole grain roll

1 teaspoon canola margarine

1 cup fat-free or low-fat (1%) milk

DAY 4

Breakfast

¾ cup bran flakes

2 tablespoons raisins

1 cup fat-free or low-fat (1%) milk

Coffee or tea with milk and sugar, if desired

Lunch

Chicken Salad

1½ cups mixed baby greens

3 ounces cooked chicken breast, cut into strips

½ cup seedless grapes

2 tablespoons chopped walnuts

2 tablespoons low-fat dressing

1 slice whole grain bread

1 teaspoon canola margarine

1 cup fat-free or low-fat (1%) milk

Snack

1 bowl vegetable soup

1 whole wheat English muffin

1 teaspoon canola margarine

Dinner

Dinner salad

3 ounces baked salmon steak with fresh lemon juice

⅔ cup steamed brown rice

1 teaspoon canola oil or canola margarine

1 cup steamed broccoli and cauliflower

1 cup steamed carrots

1 teaspoon canola oil or canola margarine

1 slice whole grain bread

1 teaspoon canola margarine

½ cup cubed papaya

¾ cup fat-free or low-fat plain yogurt

DAY 5

Breakfast

Garden Omelet

Sauté:

½ cup diced vegetables

½ cup egg whites or egg substitute in 1 teaspoon canola oil or canola margarine

1 slice rye toast

1 teaspoon canola margarine

1 small pear

1 cup fat-free or low-fat (1%) milk

Coffee or tea with milk and sugar, if desired

Lunch

Pasta with Marinara

1 cup cooked angel hair pasta

½ cup marinara sauce with garlic and herbs

1 ounce shredded low-fat mozzarella cheese

½ cup steamed green beans

1 teaspoon canola oil or canola margarine

½ cup fresh fruit salad

1 cup fat-free or low-fat (1%) milk

Snack

1 whole grain bagel

2 tablespoons almond butter

Dinner

Dinner salad

Beef and Mushroom Stir-Fry

Sauté:

¼ cup diced onions

½ cup sliced mushrooms

½ cup broccoli

3 ounces thinly sliced beef top sirloin

in 1 teaspoon sesame oil and 2 teaspoons canola oil

⅔ cup steamed brown rice

1 cup cubed cantaloupe

1 cup fat-free or low-fat (1%) milk

DAY 6

Breakfast

¾ cup fruit and nut muesli

1 tablespoon raisins

½ cup blueberries

1 slice multigrain toast

1 cup fat-free or low-fat (1%) milk

Coffee or tea with milk and sugar, if desired

Lunch

Chicken Caesar Salad

1½ cups romaine lettuce

2 ounces cooked chicken, cut into strips

2 tablespoons low-fat Caesar dressing

1 tablespoon grated low-fat Parmesan cheese

1 multigrain roll

1 teaspoon canola margarine

½ cup cubed mango

1 cup fat-free or low-fat (1%) milk

Snack

4 low-fat whole grain crackers

1 tablespoon almond butter

Dinner

Dinner salad

Baked Fish in Foil Wrap

3 ounces sea bass

½ cup sliced carrots

1 teaspoon olive oil

1 teaspoon reduced-sodium soy sauce

2 tablespoons orange juice

½ clove garlic, minced

1 cup cooked orzo

1 teaspoon canola oil or canola margarine

½ cup steamed kale

1¼ cups cubed watermelon

1 cup fat-free or low-fat (1%) milk

DAY 7

Breakfast

¾ cup multigrain cereal

1 cup fat-free or low-fat (1%) milk

1 sliced nectarine

½ multigrain bagel

1 tablespoon natural peanut butter

Coffee or tea with milk and sugar, if desired

Lunch

Turkey Sandwich

2 slices whole grain bread

3 ounces roast turkey breast

½ cup baby spinach and sliced tomato

2 teaspoons canola mayonnaise

Spring Salad

1 cup mixed salad greens

½ cup grated carrot and cucumber

1 tablespoon vinaigrette (olive-oil based)

1 tablespoon slivered almonds

¾ cup pineapple chunks

1 cup fat-free or low-fat (1%) milk

Snack

1 small baked potato

2 tablespoons fat-free sour cream

½ cup salsa

Dinner

Dinner salad

3 ounces broiled beef tenderloin

⅔ cup steamed brown rice

1 teaspoon canola oil or canola margarine

1 cup pea pods, sautéed with 1 teaspoon olive oil

½ cup berries

1 cup fat-free or low-fat (1%) milk

8

THE EXERCISE
PRESCRIPTION

AN INTRODUCTION TO EXERCISE AND YOUR HEART

I GUARANTEE YOU THIS: If everyone in America exercised for an hour a day every day of the week, this country would have a heart-health profile radically different from the alarming one we currently have!

There has been a total revolution in the acceptance of exercise as a medical treatment over the course of my career. When I was a physician in training, heart attack patients in hospitals were restricted to 2 weeks of total bed rest! We thought exercise was harmful for cardiac patients. Of course, now we know that the exact opposite is true.

In fact, exercise is one of the most important single factors contributing to cardiovascular health. And not just because of its intrinsic (and certainly important) connection to weight loss, either. Exercise is a powerful medication in its own right, one that can actually alter your body at the metabolic level. And we now know that it can play an incredibly important role in controlling and stabilizing coronary heart disease—to the point of actually reversing damage that's already been done.

Despite this evidence, we're becoming more and more sedentary, rooted to our cars, our spectator seats, and our computers. If we want healthier hearts, we have to get up off our couches—we have to get moving!

A rallying cry for more exercise doesn't have to mean a severe or traumatic change in your life. I've found over the years that my patients tend to have a fairly overblown sense of what it means "to exercise." I think that a lot of their initial resistance to beginning a sensible physical program stems from the misguided notion that making a commitment to fitness means training for the next Ironman Triathlon. They have such unrealistic expectations of what they would need to accomplish for their exercise to "count" that they never get onto the field.

You don't need to become the buff guy who stops at your juice bar, his shirt completely soaked with sweat after a 12-mile run, or that model-thin woman who by all appearances never steps foot off the stairclimber. If you're afraid you won't ever measure up to that, stop trying and start conjuring some new images!

Consider instead a very different set of models: the older couple you see power-walking every evening after dinner; the woman who always gives her toddler a run for his money at the park; or the family that bikes into town every Sunday morning to get the newspaper. Now that's the sort of exercising that I have in mind for you—not necessarily entering the next triathlon! As long as you engage in physical activity as part of a regular routine, and as long as that activity is keeping your heart rate up (more about that in a minute), that's all you need to do to reap the unique and tremendously effective cardiovascular benefits of exercise.

EXERCISE SELLS ITSELF: THE CALIFORNIA HIGHWAY PATROL STORY

Gym memberships skyrocket in January and the gyms are packed full, but come February, those healthy New Year's resolutions have faded—and gym attendance with them. Why is this? I think it is because people aren't seeing the kind of results they need to keep them motivated. Why would they keep banging their heads against an immovable wall?

Once again, I see the one-size-fits-all demon at work, and with the same undesirable results. A one-dimensional approach to our bodies and health simply doesn't work. We have to start moving, yes—but we also have to start moving smarter. The medication that works for your neighbor may not be the right one for you, any more than his diet plan would necessarily be a good fit. The same is true with exercise. You're an individual with specific physiological needs, and you need a workout that's tailor-fit to your body and your specific metabolic conditions. In the following pages, I'll show you what you need to ensure that you're getting the best workout for you, and I believe that you'll start seeing some very rewarding results.

My belief is that if you're exercising and seeing positive results, then no matter what your ultimate goals are, you'll stick with it. Indeed, I'm happy to say that most of my patients do, and it isn't because they're any better or more motivated than the rest of the population. The reason they keep at it is because they feel better once they start. They shed those extra pounds. They can see—and touch!—their toes for the first time in years, and all those minor aches and pains, the backaches, the morning stiffness, the creaky hips and joints, start to subside. Their lungs are clearer, they have more energy and more stamina for their other activities, and they find that their sex life and their mood have also improved. And guess what? After exercising, their Advanced Metabolic Marker test scores are improving, too!

Exercise's dirty little secret is that it feels good, and the results feel even better. Here's a good example of its more addictive properties. A number of years ago, I participated in a program designed to improve the cardiovascular health of the California Highway Patrol officers, who were suffering an astonishing rate of cardiovascular disease. Under the leadership of Dr. Ed Bernauer at the University of California, Davis, we put a program in place that scientifically determined how fit an officer needed to be to adequately fulfill his job requirements. What does it take to drive a car in a high-speed chase, stop, chase a suspect on foot, climb a 6-foot fence, and then wrestle the suspect to the ground? These activities were scientifically measured, a physical fitness equation was developed, and each officer had to meet these new physical requirements on an annual basis. My hidden plan was to improve cardiovascular health through physical fitness. At first, the program was met with a lot of grumbling by the officers in the field. But it worked! The cardiovascular disease rate dropped in a very satisfying way, but that's not even the point of the story: I later heard that the program had become so appreciated that officers were willing to sacrifice other benefits during a labor negotiation in order to keep it in place! And if you look at the California Highway Patrol, you won't find a fat one in the whole bunch.

People who exercise tend to live more healthfully in general: They eat better and they're less stressed out. And they look better, even if they don't drop weight—trust me, 175 pounds of muscle looks a lot better than 175 pounds of flab. So once I've gotten someone to begin, I don't have to worry about them backsliding—exercise, the type that fits your profile, sells itself.

It's for this reason that I recommend above all else that you enjoy the exercise you do. It should be a time that you look forward to, so much so that you'll sacrifice other things when necessary to do it. Make it fun, and you'll make it a habit. When your exercise program is tailor-fit to your cardiovascular type, you're going to see results. I can give you the tools to ensure that you're working out smart instead of hitting a brick wall. And while I can't stand over you while you lace up your running shoes every morning, I can give you a lot of very good, scientifically based reasons to stick with an exercise program. In other words, I think the best way to persuade you to exercise is to take a minute to convince you that exercise works.

So let's take a look at the ways that exercising can change your actual metabolic makeup.

EXERCISE AND YOUR METABOLIC PROFILE

Your heart is a muscle, and like any other muscle, the harder you work it, the stronger it gets. But there are other underlying benefits to be achieved from exercise as well. How exactly does exercise affect your metabolism and your heart? How can you use this powerful tool to strengthen your cardiovascular system at the cellular level?

First, exercise is intimately linked to weight loss, and that's one of the reasons it's so important for establishing heart health. Moreover, the actual act of exercising has a significant effect on the way that specific lipoproteins are metabolized in your body, and this process can improve some of the underlying metabolic issues that may be putting you at risk for coronary heart disease. Let's take a closer look.

Exercise and Weight Loss

As you have almost undoubtedly heard, obesity is a serious—and rapidly growing—medical epidemic in the United States, and it is one of the clearest contributing factors to our nation's high rate of coronary heart disease. We've already examined weight loss from the perspective of diet and nutrition, but it's also a crucial line item in the argument for consistent exercise.

Obesity and your level of physical activity are clearly linked—and the research on this isn't new. In 1939, a Dr. Green investigated 200 overweight adults and discovered that the onset of obesity could be traced to a sudden decrease in physical activity. Dr. Bruch, in 1940, found that 76 percent of obese boys and 88 percent of obese girls were physically inactive. Later investigators discovered that inactivity was a more important factor in obesity than overeating. And in 1960, Chiroco and Stunkard used a pedometer to discover that obese individuals move less during the day than the nonobese.

So people who move more weigh less—that's pretty well-established. But why? And how does exercise actually promote the loss of excess weight?

It works in two ways, actually. The first is the classic: Exercise promotes weight loss by helping you to burn more calories than you take in.

One of the ways that the individualized Exercise Plans are broken down is by the number of calories they burn. Calories are merely a measure of energy. The number of calories in a food indicates how much energy it will give you; the number of calories burned by an activity indicates how much energy is used when you do that activity.

There's a reason for that: The big studies on coronary heart disease stabilization and regression have used the number of calories burned as their primary unit of measurement. But if weight loss is a priority for you, you can also use your Prescription as a way to make sure that you're burning slightly more calories (about 500 a day) than you consume. This, combined with a healthy diet, is a terrific way to help you lose excess weight.

Beware: Appetite Surge!

If you're trying to lose weight and you've started an exercise program to help you do that, you're going to have to watch your calorie intake as well. Contrary to popular belief, exercising doesn't give you carte blanche to eat whatever you want.

In fact, you're going to want to be extra conscious of the calories you're eating for the first little while. When you start to exercise, you'll see that the body compensates for the energy spent exercising by looking for more fuel, which often means an increase in appetite. Studies have shown that people will replace the calories they burn by unconsciously eating different types of food, and that they actually change what they eat—lowering fat and increasing carbohydrates—without realizing that's where their cravings are taking them. If you do want to lose weight, you'll have to be very careful to stay on top of your diet, to make sure that you're not spoiling all your hard work at the gym by unconsciously increasing your caloric intake.

Don't worry, you won't have to go hungry. You just have to satisfy the craving for calorie-dense foods like sugary snacks, sweets, and sodas with healthier, less calorically weighted ones, like fruits, vegetables, and whole grain products.

For some, the opposite happens when they begin to exercise! Regular exercise in some individuals is associated with reduced appetite, so you may find that you're not only burning more calories, but also consuming less, with little or no effort.

What if I don't want to lose weight?

If you're at an ideal, lean weight and you don't want to lose any more, that doesn't mean that you shouldn't reap the metabolic benefits of exercise.

If you want to stay exactly the same lean weight but need to raise your HDL, for instance, exercise can help you do it. (Exercise is most powerful in raising HDL-C in people who have excess body fat or elevated blood triglycerides, but it's beneficial for everybody.) All you have to do is increase your healthy calories to make up for the ones you burn when you exercise. If you're burning 2,000 calories a week in your workouts, then all you have to do is supplement your diet with an additional 2,000 calories over the course of that week. But what you eat counts. Try to make up the difference with whole grains, fruits and vegetables, and low-fat dairy.

Even if you maintain a balance between the calories you take in and the calories you burn, the exercise will positively change your body fat content and distribution. In other words, you may gain lean body mass (muscle) and lose fat body mass (your love handles), so that although your body weight hasn't changed, your muscle-to-fat proportion has. You'll look and feel better even though you haven't lost a pound.

Let's look now at the impact of exercise on your actual metabolic profile for insight into the other way that exercise contributes to weight loss—and more.

Exercise, LPL, and the Triglyceride Story

Exercise also has a profound effect on the way your body's metabolism works: Working out actually makes your body more efficient. And when it comes to improving your metabolic profile through exercise, the star player at work is an enzyme called **lipoprotein lipase**, or LPL.

LPL is like a furry lining attached to the inside of your arteries. As the blood passes through, it rubs up against that hairy lining, and a number of processes occur. Most importantly, this enzyme determines how fast your body chews up triglycerides. If the LPL enzyme is working well and efficiently, your body is chewing up fats in the bloodstream very quickly; if it's not, there are going to be a lot of them floating around your system. People with elevated blood triglycerides often have LPL that isn't working as well as it should.

So here are some of the benefits of exercise at the cellular level.

First, exercise sends a message to up-regulate, or increase production, of

LPL. Because your body anticipates the need for more energy, which it gets from triglycerides, it creates more LPL to help it metabolize the triglycerides. The more LPL you produce, the faster you pull fats from your bloodstream.

We tested this hypothesis in the lab in what we called the Egg McMuffin stress test. In this test, you eat an Egg McMuffin, and we test your triglycerides a couple of hours later. Then you come back the next day after working out for an hour, and you are again given an Egg McMuffin to eat. Just like the day before, we test your triglycerides a couple of hours after you've eaten. Your post-McMuffin triglycerides will be *lower* on the second day. That means that a *single* workout has increased the speed at which your body is able to remove triglycerides from your circulation. The exercise you've done— even just that single session—has actually increased your body's efficiency at removing fats from the bloodstream.

Unfortunately, the effects are relatively short term and don't last forever. And I'm certainly not suggesting that a single bout of exercise can combat the damage done by repeated bouts of eating, drinking, and making merry. In fact, the benefits of that exercise-induced increased LPL production are optional for approximately 23 hours after exercise. This is one important reason why it makes sense for people who are trying to control high triglycerides to work out *every* day.

There are also long-term metabolic benefits to a regular exercise program. It turns out that if you exercise regularly, there's a cumulative gain. This is why a marathon runner's triglyceride count will be dramatically lower after that Egg McMuffin stress test than it would be in someone who doesn't exercise. Because he makes constant demands on his energy stores by exercising regularly, the runner has trained his body to metabolize fat more efficiently. If he were to stop running regularly, his metabolism would eventually slow down again.

Being Fat Makes You Fatter

The benefits of LPL make it even more important to maintain a healthy weight. There is a high concentration of this LPL enzyme in fat and muscle cells. Adults have all the fat cells they're ever going to have. So when you get fat, you don't actually gain more fat cells—the ones you have just get fatter. The problem with this is that when fat cells get bigger, the LPL associated with them changes shape, and then it doesn't work as efficiently. LPL is an enzyme, and the most common metaphor used to describe an enzyme is a key that causes a certain reaction to happen when it's put in the right lock. When your fat cells expand, the shape of the LPL changes. Often, when you knock a tooth off a key, or bend it, you can still make it work in the lock, but not as quickly and smoothly as before. When LPL changes, it too becomes a less efficient key.

And since LPL pulls fats from the bloodstream, you really want this enzyme to be working at peak efficiency. So at a metabolic level, whatever excess weight you're carrying is actually causing you to get even fatter! When overweight people lose weight, their fat cells get smaller, and this enzyme begins working more efficiently again. Although you haven't increased the amount of it that you have, the amount you have works better. In the long term, then, exercise encourages weight loss, which increases the efficiency of LPL, the enzyme that breaks down fat in the blood.

As you'll see later on, LPL is at the heart of many of the cardiac benefits that can be achieved through exercise.

In the next two sections, I'll walk you through what you need to know to embark on an exercise routine that can turn your heart health around. We'll start with some basics (don't skip them, even if you're a pro!), and I'll teach you how to approximate your own personal target heart rate. This will allow you to get your own best workout every time. No matter what activity you're doing or where you're doing it, you'll never feel that you're wasting time in the gym again! Then you'll be ready to be outfitted with the individualized workout plan devised especially for your metabolic profile.

EXERCISE BASICS

Before I launch you into a calorie-melting, heart-healing workout, there are some basics you need to know. I realize that many of you have not engaged in a formal exercise routine for a long time—in some cases not since you were in school! So the first thing I want to do is congratulate you. You have already taken the first and most important step just by making this commitment to your heart health.

BEGINNING AN EXERCISE PROGRAM

Remember, even if you were very athletic earlier in your life, getting started again can be a humbling—and even dangerous—experience if you don't take proper precautions. So don't push yourself, start slow, and work gradually toward your goals. Just as a prescription for a new medication must take the particulars of your medical history into account, the same is true with an exercise Prescription. There's no sense in undermining the very positive cardiac potential of exercise by sidelining yourself through careless injury or burnout, so make sure to read these recommendations before you move on to finding your personal Exercise Prescription.

Note: It is very important for you to check with your personal physician before beginning any new exercise program.

Here's a "getting started" checklist to review as you begin warming up the engine.

- Know your physical limitations.
- Increase activities of daily living.
- Pick an activity you'll love.
- Go low impact.

Know Your Physical Limitations

Before you begin your exercise program (or any other therapy path, for that matter), you should talk to your doctor. This is doubly important if you're a person at risk for coronary heart disease, someone who has symptoms of heart disease, or someone who's overweight or severely out of shape. You and your doctor must collaborate to design an exercise program for you that will minimize your risk of event. *This isn't a step you can skip.* Otherwise, you can really put yourself at serious risk.

Most physicians (and the American College of Sports Medicine) recommend that if you're over 40 years of age and are just beginning an exercise program, you should take a treadmill test to make sure that you don't have serious coronary artery blockage or another form of severe coronary heart disease. Why? So that you don't keel over during your first jog around the block. I'm not being facetious; exercise puts added strain on the heart, and you have to be careful if you're not used to it.

Several studies have tried to evaluate the risk of exercise and heart attack–related deaths. A 1999 study found that 56 percent of exertion-associated deaths in men with coronary artery disease occurred in sedentary men who engaged in sudden strenuous activity. Fourteen percent of these occurred when they were mowing the lawn. And another 14 percent occurred during sexual intercourse. There's some kind of conclusion to be drawn there, but I'll leave that to you. . . .

So you have to know that your heart is up to the challenge in a medical setting before you can safely put it to the test at the track. Your doctor will tell you if he thinks you should take some kind of stress test before beginning an exercise program, but it is absolutely something that you should discuss with him before you strenuously exert yourself.

I cannot emphasize this next point strongly enough: If you feel unwell or experience any serious discomfort while you are exercising—regardless of the kind of shape you're in or your fitness level—discontinue the exercise and call your doctor immediately. Jim Fixx, who wrote best-selling books that popularized recreational running in America, died of a heart attack during a routine run near his home. His coronary arteries were severely blocked, and it is believed that he must have been training in spite of chest pain. If so, it was a mistake that contributed to his premature death.

The next step, and this is also something you can ask your doctor to help you with, is to determine whether or not you have any physical limitations to consider when you're planning an exercise program. Again, the point of this book is not to supplant your doctor, but to augment your relationship with him.

And your doctor may very well want to have a hand in crafting your program, especially if you do have certain significant physical conditions. Someone with severe arthritis in his hands might have difficulty handling free weights, whereas someone with chronic knee injuries might want to stay away from high-impact exercise, like running or step aerobics. Bear in mind that physical limitations aren't get-out-of-jail-free cards. Sports medicine has answers to almost all of them, but you need to know what you can and can't do before you get into a situation where you're likely to injure yourself.

Increase Activities of Daily Living

No doubt some of you are worried that you're too out of shape, too busy, too unathletic, or too unmotivated to stick with a new fitness program, even if you know it's going to have a profound benefit on your heart. Don't worry.

I know that beginning an exercise program can be very daunting, especially if it's been a long time (and a lot of pounds) since your last attempt to get into shape. Your body isn't used to the activity, and it can be uncomfortable at first. But if you stick with it, starting gently and increasing the activity level very gradually, you will begin to notice it becoming easier. Your doctor may also have told you that you're too out of shape to start a rigorous exercise program immediately. I'd like to encourage you with the same advice: Work into it gently.

One way to kick-start a workout program slowly is by increasing what's called the activities of daily living—in other words, start moving in your everyday life. These things don't have to take a lot of time or effort. Park your car in a spot at the very back of the lot when you go shopping. Walk to the corner store instead of driving to the supermarket. Walk up the stairs to your office instead of taking the elevator.

Like everything else, exercise will be an easier pill to swallow if you move into it gradually. A 10-minute walk after dinner isn't so impossible, and you can gradually add time to that walk until you're walking long enough to reap even greater cardiovascular benefits. If you start with a 10-minute walk every day and increase it by 5 minutes every week, you'll be walking a total of 60 minutes in 2 or 3 months. That's a drop in the bucket when we consider that you're beginning a lifelong journey to incorporate physical activity into your life. Easing into exercise will help reduce the chance of joint, bone, and muscle injury by slowly accommodating your body (and your mind!) to routine physical activity.

Pick an Activity You'll Love

Once you're ready to begin an exercise program, your next step is to figure out the kinds of things you *like* to do. This might sound reductive or silly, but it's not. I'm asking you to make a permanent lifestyle change, to start to build habits around activities that you can happily do for the rest of your life. The biggest reason that people backslide on their exercise regimens is because they haven't thought seriously enough about the enjoyment they get from the actual activity. It's very easy to say that you'll run 5 miles every day, but if you hate every minute of it, you're going to be couch surfing in a month.

If you can bring the play back into your exercise life, then you'll reduce boredom and increase your enjoyment, and that means you'll be more likely to do it.

Go Low Impact

If you're just starting an exercise program or if you have physical limitations, you'll probably want to stick with low-impact exercise. When you jump up and down, you put a lot of stress on your joints. Low-impact exercise enables you to get your heart rate up without putting that stress on the body. It's perfect for those with joint problems or arthritis or for people who are overweight. Swimming is the ideal low-impact exercise because the body is totally cushioned by the water; there's minimal stress on the joints.

But it's possible to get a good low-impact workout on dry land as well. Walking is low impact, and even a salsa aerobics class can be made low impact with just a few modifications. A good rule of thumb: An exercise is low impact if you have one foot on the ground at all times. So instead of doing a jumping jack, you move your arms over your head the way you would nor-

WATER: HYDRATE THYSELF!

Almost everyone can afford to drink more water. It's especially easy to become volume depleted when you're exercising unless you make a conscious effort to stop and drink more water.

If you're starting an exercise program, remember to drink extra water to make up for what you're losing. This is doubly true if you live at a high altitude (or if you travel to one). Good hydration is also especially important if you're on medication. When you get dehydrated, your blood volume goes down, which means that the concentration of the medication in your bloodstream can be increased. This can worsen side effects, sometimes dramatically and with dangerous consequences. Dehydration is also one of the leading causes of constipation, which is one of the side effects of many of the heart drugs. Drinking more water can help to ease your discomfort and can also help if you've adopted a higher-fiber diet.

I encourage my patients to remind themselves to drink three *extra* large glasses of water a day, in addition to the water they'd ordinarily drink: one big glass in the morning, one in the afternoon, and one in the evening. Caffeinated beverages, like coffee, tea, soda, or performance-enhancing beverages like Jolt and Red Bull don't count, either—caffeine is a diuretic and will in fact increase your dehydration. If you're dying for something with a little more pizzazz, drink fizzy water with a little lemon or lime squeezed in.

mally, but move one leg out to the side at a time instead of hopping out with both. Most aerobics exercises can be modified in this way.

Once you've gotten your doctor's okay and you've started to think about some low-impact activities that you're likely to enjoy over the long run, it's time to figure out how you can personalize your workouts to get the best results possible.

DETERMINING *YOUR* TARGET HEART RATE

At the heart of my cardiac health program is a move away from an overly standardized, one-size-fits-all approach, and the Exercise Prescription is no exception. We can now individualize exercise plans to work specifically for your particular cardiac profile.

One of my pet peeves is those charts, so common in fitness magazines, that list the number of calories burned during common exercises. It's simply not scientific; there's too much wiggle room. How many calories you burn doing anything depends on how hard you work. Yes, it's totally possible to burn 300 calories an hour playing tennis. It's also possible to burn 80—if you don't lift your feet. Or 150 if you play hard but take two 10-minute breaks.

I'm concerned that these charts are misleading. People get unmotivated if they don't see results. If you're expecting the benefits of a 300-calorie workout but you're only burning 80 calories, no wonder you're not thrilled with your outcome! It's not that exercise doesn't work—it's just that you need to exercise more efficiently.

There's a simple way for you to escape the frustration of an 80-calorie workout dressed up like a 300-calorie workout, and it's one that you can take with you wherever you go. I'm referring, of course, to your **target heart rate**, or your **heart rate training zone**. This simple calculation provides you with a way to tell for sure, and without any fancy equipment, how hard and how consistently you're working.

Think of target heart rate as the "dose" of this Exercise Prescription. Telling someone to "play volleyball" is a bit like telling him to take "some" fenofibrate. You don't take an unspecified amount of a coronary heart disease drug, you take a specific dosage. When your doctor prescribes 200 milligrams of fenofibrate, there's a very good, patient-specific reason it's not 150 milligrams, or 400. Exercise should work the same way. If you work out for 30 minutes with your heart rate at 100 beats per minute, you're getting a less intense "dose" than if you'd kept your heart rate at 140 beats per minute, because 140 beats per minute is a higher "dose."

Everyone's target heart rate is different, and we'll show you how to calculate yours. In the Nutrition Prescription, I gave you the tools to determine your precise caloric needs so you could get away from standardized calorie requirements. In the same way, once you know what your target heart rate should be, you can get away from those loosey-goosey fitness "recommendations" and into an exercise program that works for *you*—not an idealized, population-based average of "people sort of like you."

Your target heart rate is the heart rate you want to maintain throughout your workout. That target range is between 60 and 80 percent of your **maximum heart rate**. Here's how you can calculate your own personal target heart rate.

Step One: Find Your Resting Heart Rate

In order to find your **resting heart rate** (RHR), you'll take your pulse when you first wake up in the morning or after 5 minutes of total rest and relaxation. No matter how you take this measure, it is important that you do it the same way every time—and that means that if you swing your legs over and sit on the edge of your bed when you're testing it, you should do it that way the next time. I suggest that you take it every morning for 3 days and average the results. That's your RHR.

Step Two: Find Your Maximum Heart Rate

You'll also need to know your **maximum heart rate (MHR)**, the highest heart rate that you can safely achieve. The best way to get your MHR, especially if you're overweight, out of shape, have a family history of coronary heart disease, or are a cardiac patient, is from a treadmill stress test, which is given *only* under the supervision of a physiologist, nurse, or physician.

An age-predicted MHR is easier to obtain and relatively accurate if you're in good health. It can be calculated by subtracting your age from 220. (I would always prefer and recommend that you do the stress test under professional supervision so you're not relying on any guesswork!)

> 220 − your age = your MHR

The maximum heart rate for James, a 55-year-old, is 220 − 55, or 165 beats per minute [bpm]). That means that James's heart shouldn't beat more than 165 times per minute (or more than 28 beats every 10 seconds).

Step Three: Find Your Heart Rate Reserve

Next, you subtract your resting heart rate (RHR) from your maximum heart rate (MHR) to establish your **heart rate reserve** (HRR). So,

$$MHR - RHR = HRR$$

James's resting heart rate is 60 bpm. We know that his MHR is 165, so his HRR is 165 − 60, or 105.

Step Four: Find Your Target Heart Rate Range

Your target heart rate is really a range. So we'll use a multiplier to determine the low and high ends of your target range, or training zone. To find the low end, multiply your heart rate reserve (HRR) by 60 percent (0.6) and add your resting heart rate (RHR):

$$([MHR - RHR] \times 0.6) + RHR = \text{the low end of your target heart rate}$$

And to find the high end, multiply your heart rate reserve by 80 percent (0.8):

$$([MHR - RHR] \times 0.8) + RHR = \text{the upper end of your target heart rate}$$

This is called the **Karvonen equation,** and it gives you the heart rate range you should be exercising in. (The results can be divided by 6 to discover the number of beats every 10 seconds.)

The low end of James's target heart rate, then, is (105 × 0.6) + 60, or 123 bpm (or 20 beats every 10 seconds). The high end of his target heart rate is (105 × 0.8) + 60, or 144 bpm (or 24 beats every 10 seconds).

As long as James's heart is beating between 123 and 144 beats per minute for the duration of his workout, he's maximizing the cardiac benefit he's getting from every minute he exercises. This range is his heart rate training zone.

How to Check Your Heart Rate

Checking your heart rate while you're exercising is pretty simple. Use your fingers (never your thumb!) to feel for your pulse, either at your neck or at your wrist, and count the number of beats you feel for 10 seconds. Multiply the number of beats you get by six to come up with the number of beats per minute.

Many gym machines have ways to monitor your heart rate; in fact, on many of them, you can plug in your desired range, and it'll beep if you go above or below that range. If you're exercising outdoors, you can also buy a very inexpensive heart rate monitor at most sporting-goods stores. These are simple to use: You wrap a strap around your chest, which measures your heart rate, and you can check the results on a digital readout that you wear on your wrist like a watch.

Another way that physiologists and cardiologists measure exertion is with something called a Borg scale, which assigns a numeric value to the amount of perceived exertion, measured by how difficult it is for a patient to exercise: 1 is very light; 20 is maximum exertion.

Shortness of breath is another pretty reliable indicator of exertion level and heart rate and is easier to check while you're exercising than counting your pulse is. You can easily modify this test for your own purposes; your breath should be coming fast during your workout, but you should always be able to complete a full sentence. If you can't complete one full sentence, you're probably working too hard and entering the anaerobic zone, which means you're not getting enough oxygen to your cells. If you can complete *two* full sentences, you may not be not working hard enough and need to increase the intensity slightly.

The Benefits of Monitoring Your Heart Rate

It's important to monitor your heart rate and to stay within your target range the *whole time* you're working out or you risk wasting your time (if you're under your target) or hurting yourself (if you're over it). I've had a number of patients come in to see me over the years, complaining that they "can't" lose weight or change their blood work results, despite their daily exercise programs. "I spend hours on the treadmill, and I haven't lost a pound!" they say. Often, these people simply aren't working hard enough. They're not getting—and keeping—their heart rates up.

It's not enough to amble around the park or to lean on your golf club while your buddy lines up his shot. It's probably better for you than watching a *Law & Order* rerun, but it's not real exercise. I want to make this very clear: Exercise is a different animal entirely. You should enjoy what you're doing, yes, but you have to work reasonably hard to see results. And one of the best ways to tell how hard you're working is to measure your heart rate.

One hour of exercise in the Exercise Prescription generally means an hour of continuous exercise with your heart rate in your training zone—between the low and high ends of your target heart rate range. You can speed up and slow down, but you should stay within that training zone to achieve optimal results.

Remember, you're just trying to keep your heart rate within the range, and you'll be surprised at how easy it is to hit and maintain that lower level. Your heart doesn't have to be going like gangbusters the whole time. Running like a bat out of hell isn't going to do you much good if you're only doing it for 15 minutes *and* it's stressful for your body.

Athletes often train in **intervals**, which means that they alternate between varying levels of intensity—running for 4 minutes, walking briskly for 3, and then repeating the cycle, for example. Their heart rate seldom goes below the low end of the desired target, but the lower-intensity segments allow them to train longer without excessive fatigue. So if you stretch that horrible, heart-pounding 15-minute run out over 45 minutes, walking briskly between the intervals, you're actually getting a better workout—and one that's considerably more enjoyable to boot.

The real benefit of working out using your target heart rate is that you can do *anything*, and I think you'll find that this frees you up considerably. You can trim the hedges, you can swing dance, you can swim, run, walk, cycle, box—or a million other options. As long as your heart rate stays within the desired range for the prescribed amount of time, you're getting the job done.

Now that we've covered the basics, let's get down to the business of getting you outfitted for your Exercise Prescription!

THE EXERCISE PLANS

My patients know that when I talk to them about the importance of exercise to their hearts, I mean it. They know because I ask about it every single time I see them. And every single time, I let them know that exercise isn't something they should do if they feel like it or get the chance. It's indispensable, not an add-on.

I consider exercise a part of their treatment, and I expect them to comply in the same way that I expect them to remember to take their medication. In this way, I make them see that the exercise "prescription" is as essential a component of their therapy as any medication I might also prescribe.

In order to underscore this message we have an "exercise prescription pad" in the clinic that looks exactly like a regular prescription pad. On it, instead of writing "200 milligrams of fenofibrate, once a day, every day. Possible side effect: GI distress," I'll write something more along these lines: "Jogging, 60 minutes, daily, at a heart rate of 110 beats per minute. Possible side effect: You may eventually need to buy smaller pants." Just like a drug prescription, an exercise prescription should include the type, intensity, duration, and frequency of the medication.

That's just one example—you certainly don't have to jog if you're more comfortable doing something else! But the Prescription metaphor helps me to get across an important point: Exercise is like a heart medication in two important ways.

First of all, like medication, exercise *works*, and it works well. In fact, it can be as effective as some of the most potent medicines out there. My new patients are constantly astounded to discover what a profound and direct effect a regular exercise program can have on their cardiovascular systems. They come back into my office trim and fit and waving their new numbers, as amazed as if they were the first one ever. And I never, ever say "I told you so" because, in truth, they deserve the credit. But I'm not surprised by their terrific results.

Secondly, as with drugs, the beneficial effects of exercise have a limited half-life. That means they only exist in the body's system for a certain amount of time. If you're on medication, you have to take that medication every day because the drug is only powerful for so long. In order to keep experiencing the benefits, you will eventually need another dose. And drugs with a limited half-life have to be taken twice a day or in a time-release formula.

Exercise also has a limited half-life—its fantastic benefits, which we'll discuss fully in this chapter, only last for a certain amount of time in your system. This is why we recommend daily exercise as the best-possible-case scenario. That way, you're never without those benefits.

So, just like a drug prescription does, the following Exercise Prescriptions define the **type**, **intensity**, **duration**, and **frequency** of the medication involved. Let's take a look at what each of those entails before we prescribe the individualized plan that fits your cardiac profile.

TYPE OF EXERCISE

The type of exercise we're talking about in this section is **endurance exercise**, which means it involves repetitive movement of the large muscle groups in the body for an extended amount of time.

The Exercise Plans will leave you free to fill in the blanks in terms of what *type* of endurance exercise you prefer. The freedom to choose what you enjoy most is the key to keeping you on the program! The whole point is for you to have fun with it. Obviously, there are literally dozens of ways to get endurance exercise. It seems that every day, a gym is announcing a new way to get in shape, but don't forget the tried and true favorites: walking, running, swimming, cycling, and strength training.

These are just some of the many endurance exercise options available to you. Look around your community and find your own! There are martial-arts classes, flow-style yoga classes, dance classes, stairclimbers, elliptical trainers, all different kinds of sports—in short, whatever gets you moving is the right type of "medicine" for our Exercise Prescription.

INTENSITY OF EXERCISE

As I discussed in detail in the last chapter, establishing and maintaining a target heart rate is one of the best and most scientific ways to determine that your workouts are of sufficient intensity for your heart to receive exercise's beneficial effects—the correct dosage, in other words, personalized for you. This is a key ingredient if you want to see results—it's essential to make sure that you're working within your target heart rate training zone for the pre-scribed number of minutes. If you're not, you're not getting your medica-tion—it's like taking half a pill.

I think you'll be pleasantly surprised to see how easy it is to get your heart rate into that target training zone. You don't have to run like a cheetah for hours and hours to see great results! On page 220, we talked about training in intervals, which allows you to alternate periods of high exertion with lower exertion. Obviously, the harder you work, the greater the benefits, but don't go above the high end of your target range.

Working within your target heart rate training zone is not only a much more individualized way to work, but it also gives you a tremendous amount of freedom. Now that you can calculate your own personal heart rate, you can work out any way you want to. You can go for a run—10,000 miles away from the treadmill at home that calculates the number of calories you've burned—and you'll still know that you've gotten a terrific workout. You can play touch football with your kids, go for a hike, or swing dance the night away! Having this tool not only personalizes your Exercise Prescription, but it gives you tremendous latitude in designing a workout that you can live with over the long haul.

DURATION OF EXERCISE

One of the best studies on the effect of exercise on coronary heart disease was the Heidelberg Regression Study, which used a low-fat diet and lots of exercise to see a reduction in arteriographic progression—a rollback in the amount of perceptible coronary heart disease.

The results were clear: People who burned 1,000 calories a week through exercise saw their disease progress. People who burned 1,500 calories a week through exercise stabilized their disease, and people who burned 2,200 calories a week or more actually saw regression. To burn 2,200 calories a week, you have to do approximately an hour of endurance activity 7 days a week. And no drugs were used in this study—just a good diet and regular exercise.

Here's one of the major mistakes that people make when they're working out and one of the primary reasons they don't see the results they want. "I went for a 20-minute run" is certainly better than staying home and warming the couch, but it's missing a central ingredient, and that's *duration*. Twenty minutes isn't really long enough to see appreciable results.

The Heidelberg study is the basis for the Exercise Prescriptions that I have devised for you. Over the years I have "replicated" its results over and over in the patients I work with—and I can tell you that those that work out for an hour a day see fantastic results. Make sure you follow the duration portion of your specific Exercise Prescription, and make sure to keep your heart rate in your training zone for a minimum of half an hour.

FREQUENCY OF EXERCISE

Does it matter how often you exercise, as long as you're burning the recommended number of calories?

There are really two answers to that question. In the major studies that have been done, an improvement in cardiovascular health has been correlated to the number of calories burned in a week. So that would seem to indicate that the answer is no, although I would certainly not recommend that you

WARM UP AND COOL DOWN

I'd like all of you to add 10 minutes onto your workout—5 minutes on each end—to warm your body up and to cool it down.

These are important steps. It's very unsettling for your body to be thrown into serious physical activity with no warning and without any preparation. We're animals, after all. Your body can't really differentiate between different kinds of running: the kind you do on the treadmill at Bally's and the kind you do when you're being chased by a bear. So when you start your workout by launching right into working at 75 percent of your maximum heart rate, it's an extremely stressful event for the body.

Your warm-up doesn't have to be elaborate—just do what feels good. Start moving the major muscle groups and the major joints. Do some head rolls, some arm circles, some gentle squats. Sports physiologists are divided on whether stretching prevents injury, but it certainly improves performance and feels good, so stretch the major muscle groups gently before you start: Hold some lunges, touch your toes, reach side to side. Your body will tell you which areas are tight and need attention.

When you start your activity, start slowly, and you'll actually be able to feel your muscles warming up. Allow your heart rate to climb gradually into the target zone.

The same thing is true for cooling down. You want to gently lower your heart rate down from its elevated state to its resting state. So for the last 5 minutes of your workout, start concentrating on slowing down. You want to keep moving, giving your heart rate the chance to drop back naturally. If you were running, walk—first briskly and then more slowly. Walking is a good cooldown after any exercise. Even marching in place or walking around the playing field a couple of times will do the trick.

End your workout with a few stretches while your muscles are still warm. This is actually the best time to get all the benefits of stretching, and you'll be gratified to see how much more flexible you are than when you started.

work out any less than three separate sessions a week. Three times a week should really be considered the minimum required to maintain basic physical function.

Exercise *Every* Day: A General Recommendation

In fact, I recommend daily exercise for optimal results because I believe that there's good science to support that recommendation. The benefits that we reap from exercise: a reduction in platelet stickiness, for example, increased LPL activity, or the overall increase in your metabolic rate—these benefits all last about 24 hours after the workout. So if you want to continue to benefit from them all the time, it stands to reason that you'd exercise every day.

In the clinic, we analyze each patient's schedule to figure out how they can best and most comfortably fit a regular exercise program into their lives. There's no point in setting a schedule that's impossible for someone to meet, and there's no point in them feeling guilty about a missed workout if it's always impossible. If Saturday is a family day for you, then skip your jog. If Wednesdays are always busy at work, then don't break your back getting to the gym: Just make sure you work out well on Tuesday and Thursday. Five times a week is still terrific, and if you can incorporate some real activity—a long walk at lunch or a game of catch after dinner—into your "days off," that's even better.

And again, I want to encourage you to make the activities pleasurable. Mix up the types of exercise you do in a week so you don't get bored, and do things you like! And you'll find that you get better at incorporating exercise into your everyday life the longer you do it and the fitter you get—maybe you can go in-line skating with your kids instead of skipping your Saturday workout entirely.

FINDING YOUR EXERCISE PRESCRIPTION

My goal with these exercise programs is not to help you build beautiful-looking muscles or to give you rippling six-pack abs—although those may be some welcome "side effects." These exercise programs are therapeutic tools to help treat the metabolic disorders identified in your Advanced Metabolic Marker tests.

If you're going to use exercise as a tool to fight coronary heart disease the way you'd use a drug, you have to use the right "dose" and take your medicine with the correct frequency. As with the Nutrition, Medication, and Supplement components of this program, you'll use the Prescription Key on page 228 to help you locate the individualized Exercise Plan that has been calibrated to meet the needs of your particular cardiac profile. All you'll need to do is match the results of your own tests against the Prescription Key to find the plan that is right for you.

Our first Exercise Plan, **Low Dose: The Stamina Buildup Plan**, is for those of you who are are just getting started, who haven't yet gotten your metabolic marker results, or who have a very low risk of cardiac disease—the perfect low dose to either start you up or to ensure that you don't get detrained due to inadequate physical activity. Plan #2, **Your Magic Bullet: The Conversion Plan**, is especially for LDL pattern Bs. This condition puts you at such high risk that I designed a workout that will in fact use exercise to change the type of lipoprotein your body produces. The third plan, which we call **Mega-Dose: The Risk-Busters Plan**, is a no-holds-barred, full-on war against coronary heart disease using exercise as a weapon and is perfect for those of you with a combination of metabolic disorders.

Using the Prescription Key

Directly below the Exercise Prescription Key on page 228 you'll see a list of four markers labeled "My Exercise Markers." These will determine which individualized Exercise Plan is the right fit for your cardiac profile.

Refer back to your Quick Reference Chart on page 91 to help you to fill in a "yes" or "no" in the space provided beside each Exercise Marker. (Let's do an example together: Jessica has tested "normal" on LDL pattern B, apo E2, insulin, and HDL2b, so her column would read "No," "No," "No," "No.")

The Exercise Prescription Key

Exercise Marker															
LDL pattern B	Yes	Yes	Yes	Yes	Yes	Yes	Yes	Yes	Yes	Yes	No	No	No	No	No
Apo E2	Yes	Yes	Yes	No	No	No	Yes	No	No	Yes	No	Yes	Yes	Yes	No
Insulin	No	No	Yes	Yes	No	No	No	Yes	Yes	No	No	Yes	Yes	No	Yes
HDL2b	No	No	No	No	Yes	Yes	Yes	Yes	Yes	No	No	Yes	No	No	No
Exercise Plan #:	2	2	3	3	3	3	3	3	3	3	1	3	2	1	2

Exercise Plan #1: Low Dose: The Stamina Buildup Plan

Exercise Plan #2: Your Magic Bullet: The Conversion Plan

Exercise Plan #3: Mega-Dose: The Risk-Busters Plan

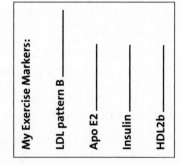

My Exercise Markers:

LDL pattern B _____

Apo E2 _____

Insulin _____

HDL2b _____

Once you have your list of yeses and no's, just look up at the Key and find the column that duplicates your pattern. (Remember, read down the columns, from top to bottom, until you find your exact match.)

At the base of the column that matches your own results, you'll find the number that identifies *your* plan. (Jessica would find the plan that matches her four "no's" in the 12th column from the left. Since the number at the base of the column is 1, she should proceed to the first Exercise Plan, Low Dose: The Stamina Buildup Plan.)

So refer back to your Quick Reference Chart on page 91, and let's get started!

Note: If you haven't taken the Advanced Metabolic Marker tests or if you're still waiting for your results, don't worry—we're not leaving you out. You should proceed directly to the first plan, Low Dose: The Stamina Buildup Plan. When your results come back (or if you decide to be tested in the future), you'll be able to insert your results into the Prescription Key as we've described above.

EXERCISE PLAN #1
LOW DOSE:
THE STAMINA BUILDUP PLAN

This is a relatively light Exercise Plan, what you might think of as a "low dose." In fact, it's the minimal amount of exercise that I'd recommend. It's just enough to keep your joints fluid and your muscles from becoming detrained. That's why I've called it the Stamina Buildup Plan—it's the first step on your fitness journey.

Who Should Use This Exercise Plan?

- People beginning an exercise program
- People without coronary heart disease
- People who have not yet taken their Advanced Metabolic Marker tests

People Beginning an Exercise Program

If you're someone who's just beginning to work out again after a long time away (or someone who's never seen the inside of a gym in your life), this is a good place for you to start.

Beginning an Exercise Plan is a lifestyle change, and as with all lifestyle changes, you're going to want to acclimatize both your body and your mind as gently as possible. Working out three times a week will help to get your muscles and cardiovascular system into shape, and you'll begin to see how you can fit exercise into your daily routine.

People without Coronary Heart Disease

You're not going to see a whole lot of cardiac benefit from this plan, which is why it's my prescription for people without existing cardiac disease and those who are at the lowest levels of risk. In this section, we're using exercise as a therapy to treat specific disorders. In the same way that I don't prescribe medicine when there's nothing wrong with a patient, this is the Exercise Plan I recommend when there's nothing to treat. It's not a powerful remedy because a powerful remedy isn't required.

That said, the benefits of exercise—as a preventive measure and as it contributes to overall health—are well-supported.

EXERCISE PLAN #1: LOW DOSE: THE STAMINA BUILDUP PLAN

- **Type:** Endurance exercise
- **Intensity:** Your target heart rate training zone
- **Duration and frequency:** 90 minutes a week. Recommended: 30 minutes, three times a week

  Burns 1,000 calories

EXERCISE PLAN #2
YOUR MAGIC BULLET: THE CONVERSION PLAN

This plan is what you might call a moderate dose of exercise. I like to think of this one as our secret weapon against the "stealth" heart attack!

Who Should Use This Exercise Plan?

- People with LDL pattern B

People with LDL Pattern B

LDL pattern B means that a high percentage of your LDL cholesterol is made up of small particles, which are very atherogenic. As you'll remember, LDL pattern B is one of the most serious metabolic conditions you can have when it comes to cardiac risk.

As serious as this condition is, there's also good news: People with LDL pattern B are extremely responsive to treatment. In particular, it has been shown that this type of LDL is exceptionally responsive to exercise! So the right exercise plan is strongly indicated for people who are LDL pattern B. In the Stanford Weight Loss Study, we were actually able to convert people, at this level of exercise, from the very atherogenic small LDL pattern B to the far safer large LDL pattern A.

How does it work?

First of all, exercise helps you lose weight, which is the first order of business for a person with LDL pattern B. It's actually easier for an overweight person to convert from LDL pattern B to LDL pattern A than for a thin person to do it. Most of the time, all an overweight person has to do is eat right, exercise, and lose weight to increase the efficiency of that all-important lipoprotein lipase (LPL) enzyme. But if you're already trim and have good habits and your LDL is still small, that may be an indication that you have a powerful genetic abnormality in the way your body handles these small LDLs. If that is the case, it will be more difficult for you to see improvement compared to the husky guy who's exercising and losing weight on the stairclimber next to yours.

However, exercise can still help a lot! This bit of magic is also linked to another enzyme—LPL's evil twin, called hepatic lipase (HL). As we know, exercise causes your body to up-regulate the production of the essential enzyme LPL. This is a good thing for two reasons. First of all, the more LPL you have, the more efficiently your body is metabolizing fat. But there's also a parallel enzyme to LPL: HL, which hangs out in the liver. Both enzymes affect the way the body chews up fats, but they have opposite effects: When HL is working efficiently, it promotes the expression of, or increases, small LDL particles. When LPL goes up, HL goes down, and when HL goes up, LPL goes down. Therefore, increasing your amount of LPL automatically suppresses HL, which decreases small LDL.

And this, too, is linked to weight loss. At Stanford University in 1985, as part of a National Institutes of Health research study, I extracted body fat from research subjects and showed that as you get fatter, LPL in the fat tissue goes down and HL goes up—but as you lose body fat, LPL goes up and HL goes down.

My own cholesterol numbers are normal, but I do have small LDL pattern B, so I make sure that I stick to my personal Exercise Plan no matter what, even when I'm very busy or traveling. It's the best way I know to control that dangerous metabolic condition!

EXERCISE PLAN #2: YOUR MAGIC BULLET: THE CONVERSION PLAN

- **Type:** Endurance exercise

- **Intensity:** Your target heart rate training zone

- **Duration and frequency:** 210 minutes a week. Recommended: Work out for 30 minutes, seven times a week, or for 70 minutes, three times a week

  Burns 1,500 calories

EXERCISE PLAN #3

MEGA-DOSE: THE RISK-BUSTERS PLAN

In this plan, the "dose"—the amount you have to exercise and how often—is higher because the number of problems you're confronting is higher. Most people will see positive results if they exercise at this level.

This plan is what you might consider a full-strength dose, what I like to think of as the full-throttle, gloves-off, take-no-prisoners fitness campaign against cardiac disease.

Who Should Use This Exercise Plan?

- People with existing coronary heart disease
- People with apo E2 in combination with another condition that raises triglycerides
- People with elevated insulin levels
- People with low HDL (the *good* cholesterol!)
- People with multiple metabolic disorders

People with Existing Coronary Heart Disease

Exercising 7 days a week for an hour at each session is my Prescription for everyone with existing coronary heart disease. The Heidelberg Regression Study, which took place in Heidelberg, Germany, is one of the most compelling arguments for daily exercise out there. In that study, without any drugs or medical intervention save daily exercise and a good diet, researchers demonstrated that you can actually see an improvement in the damage that has already been done to the heart.

So this is what it takes if you want to take your best exercise shot against the cardiac threat that's gunning for you. There's no guarantee, but it is possible that with this Exercise Prescription you can actually stall, or even reverse, the progression of the disease. Especially when it is combined with the other Prescriptions, this plan is a powerful weapon against existing coronary heart disease.

People with Apo E2

This next marker is a good example of the way that these tests give us a real preventive edge against coronary heart disease.

If you're one of the apo E2/2 people, then you know that you're at risk for type 3 hyperlipidemia, a condition that manifests itself when you don't control your triglycerides. (You can actually sometimes spot type 3 hyperlipidemia people at parties—they frequently have fatty deposits around their elbows and sometimes yellow-orange streaks, which are actually cholesterol deposits, in the creases of their palms.)

Of 100 people with type 3 hyperlipidemia, 98 percent of them have the E2/2 allele, or gene type. So this marker indicates a very strong genetic predisposition to developing this condition. But although 1 percent of people are E2/2, only 1 in 10,000 people actually expresses type 3 hyperlipidemia. In other words, only a few E2/2s present this dangerous type 3 condition—because the other 99 percent take good care of themselves by controlling their sugar and alcohol intake and their weight and by getting regular exercise.

As I've said before, this type 3 issue is a beautiful demonstration of the gene-environment interaction. These E2/2 people are genetically predisposed to develop a condition that has a very detrimental effect on their heart health. It's in their genes! But, by staying on top of their lifestyle issues—in this case, by using exercise to stimulate LPL and control their triglycerides—they duck this particular genetic bullet.

People with Elevated Insulin Levels

Exercise also improves the way your body uses insulin. As you'll remember, insulin is the chemical that helps your body to regulate the amount of sugar in your blood. When you eat a meal, your blood sugar goes up, and your body releases insulin, which allows the cells to store the sugar as potential energy. Some people are resistant to insulin, which means that the insulin is not doing an efficient job, and their blood sugar strays up.

So the body responds to this by secreting more insulin into the bloodstream in an attempt to control the blood sugar. This can go on for some time, and in this stage, it's called insulin resistance, because the body is relatively resistant to the action of the insulin and demands more to get the job done. After a while, the body's ability to make enough insulin to keep up with the demand poops out, and blood sugar begins to rise. If this continues, type 2 diabetes mellitus and all the serious adverse heart conditions associated with it develop. So for many years prior to the diagnosis of type 2 diabetes mellitus, people are insulin resistant and have higher blood levels of insulin than normal.

Like LPL, insulin simply works better when you lose that excess body fat.

You may have heard the term "butt-to-gut ratio" when people are talking about coronary heart disease risk. It's true that you're at higher risk for heart disease if you carry your excess weight around your middle, like an apple, as opposed to carrying that additional weight on your hips, rear end, and thighs, like a pear. There is a scientific reason for this, and it's linked to the connection between insulin and exercise.

There are actually two different kinds of fat stores: There's the kind that gives you a belly, and there's the kind that's stored under your skin. Think of fat as another organ, like your liver or your intestines. It has an influence on your metabolic issues, just like your other organs do.

Free fatty acids make up triglycerides, and the existence of an excess amount of these free fatty acids drives insulin production. In other words, when you have a lot of these free fatty acids in your blood, your body calls for more insulin to deal with them. Interestingly, the different fat stores respond in different ways to insulin. The fat that's stored in the belly is more insulin resistant than the kind that's stored under the skin. So the body has to keep calling for more and more insulin to deal with the fat that's stored in the belly—and that means that there's more atherogenic insulin in the bloodstream if you're heavy around the waist.

Exercise essentially works the way some diabetes drugs do: It reduces free fatty acids. For the first couple of minutes that you exercise, you're burning blood sugar, and then your body goes to the fat stores, where it converts fat into energy and burns it. Since free fatty acids are the gas that drives insulin production, those people who have a high amount of fat around their abdomens—who are more insulin resistant—have a lot to gain from eliminating these free fatty acids.

This is one of the reasons why men have been shown to reap slightly more benefit from exercise than women. As you've probably noticed, men tend to carry their excess weight around their middles, in the proverbial spare tire, whereas women tend to gain weight in their hips and thighs—a relatively less-dangerous place to store fat because it's less insulin resistant. Because men with fat around their middles are more insulin resistant, they have more to gain from burning those free fatty acids that drive insulin production.

When you don't exercise and you're insulin resistant, you crank out more insulin to deal with those excess free fatty acids. Of course, insulin is atherogenic. Insulin is also linked to problems following angioplasty because it stimulates smooth muscle growth. Your arteries are surrounded by smooth muscle, and when those smooth muscle cells replicate abnormally, they contribute to clogging up your recently opened coronary artery. So anyone with elevated levels of insulin can benefit from regular doses of exercise.

People with Low HDL

The correlation between high triglycerides and low HDL is well-documented, and that star enzyme LPL is the key to this interaction as well.

Triglycerides ride around in the blood in very low-density lipoprotein (VLDL) particles, which are like big bubbles filled with triglycerides and a little bit of cholesterol. As the VLDL particles pass through the arteries, LPL chews on the outside of these bubbles, and the triglycerides inside are released and processed into energy sources. If you're not producing enough LPL to metabolize the triglycerides, they keep riding around in the VLDL particles, which makes your blood triglyceride count really high.

But there's something else going on. There are proteins attached to the surface of these bubbles, and they're essential building blocks for the good lipoprotein, or HDL. When LPL chews at the surface of the VLDLs, these building blocks are released into the bloodstream and can be used to build

HDL. The more chewing that goes on, the more building blocks are released. So the more LPL enzyme you have, the more beneficial HDL cholesterol you'll have. That's why, when triglycerides and VLDLs are high, HDL is often low, and when triglycerides and VLDLs are low because they've all been chewed up, HDL is often high. Since exercise encourages the production of LPL, it contributes to an increase in HDL as well.

The high HDL–exercise connection was discovered in large part through a scientific accident. Dr. Peter Wood at Stanford University had been a well-respected long-distance runner in Great Britain when he was younger, and he continued to run all his life. He even established a running club for us old folks called the 50+ Runners. A few years ago, he was conducting studies on a method to measure HDL, but he couldn't find any students to draw test blood on, so he used his own and discovered that the HDL-C was ridiculously high for a man. So he drew another sample and tested it again—still wildly high. He asked himself: What's the difference between me and the students I usually use for these tests? Of course, the difference was that the students went to the movies for exercise and he ran 80 miles a week. So that's how the connection between exercise and HDL-C was first made.

And once again, weight loss comes into play. When you exercise and lose weight, your triglycerides go down and your HDL goes up. If your triglycerides are too high, then it's hard for your body to manufacture HDL. *The greatest increase in HDL is seen when exercise results in a loss of excess body fat.*

Note: Occasionally, we encounter a special group of individuals who don't see a beneficial increase in HDL through exercise. These individuals have a condition called hypoalphalipoproteinemia, a deficiency in the A1 protein, one of the surface building block proteins. In that situation, there's not a lot you can do to produce higher levels of HDL, so we tend to really hammer at LDL (the bad cholesterol) and other risk factors that we actually can do something about.

In all probability, in the future, gene therapy will be used to increase levels of HDL. In promising studies at the University of California, Dr. Ed-

EXERCISE PLAN #3: MEGA-DOSE: THE RISK-BUSTERS PLAN

- **Type:** Endurance exercise

- **Intensity:** Your target heart rate training zone

- **Frequency and duration:** 420 minutes a week. Recommended: Work out for 60 minutes, seven times a week

  Burns 2,000 calories

ward Rubin has now successfully shown that mice can be *cured* of coronary heart disease with a single injection of a gene that up-regulates the body's production of HDL. Until recently, these experiments had been restricted to animals, but Dr. P. K. Shah in Los Angeles has now conducted very early studies in humans and the results look promising for humans in the future! In the meantime, keep exercising. Most people will see an increase in HDL, and even those who don't will gain other significant benefits.

MAINTAINING YOUR RESULTS

Like everything else, you have to stay on top of your exercise program by watching your results and by modifying your program accordingly.

Three to four months after you've embarked upon your new Exercise Plan, it is time for you to take the Advanced Metabolic Marker tests again. You and your doctor will be able to see by the results whether you are responding adequately to treatment. The good results will be visible this quickly!

If your triglycerides have come down from 300 to 70, that's perfect. Keep doing exactly what you're doing. On the other hand, if they drop only to 250, that tells your doctor that you're responding to this treatment, but not as strongly as we'd hoped you would. You need to do more in order to get greater gains and more forward progress in your treatment. As you continue your exercise program, your numbers will generally continue to improve over the next 9 months, particularly if you continue to lose excess body fat. However, you will often see the biggest change in the first 3 months—if you really get with the program.

Don't waste your energy comparing your progress to anyone else's. People are all metabolically different, and what works for the guy on the treadmill next to you won't necessarily work for you. You might have to work a little harder (or he might!) to see the same results.

You'll also need to update your workout as your body gets better at it (this is called getting into shape). It's one of the great injustices of life that the better shape you're in, the harder you have to work to see results. An efficient body burns fewer calories than an inefficient one. This has positive effects on the rest of your life: An efficient body is less tired after lifting a toddler or climbing a flight of stairs or carrying a 30-pound briefcase filled with legal documents, too. And you enjoy it more! But it means that you'll have to work a little harder to get the same results at the gym as well.

Let's cross that bridge when we come to it, shall we? For now let's just focus on getting fit so that you can deploy one of the most powerful weapons we have to fight coronary heart disease.

9

THE MEDICATION
PRESCRIPTION

AN INTRODUCTION TO MEDICATIONS AND YOUR HEART

Medications are an essential part of my doctor's bag. They're wonderful tools, ones that have the power to make my patients feel better and more able to participate meaningfully in the activities they enjoy. In many cases, they have slowed the relentless progression of coronary heart disease and added years onto lives.

Although it's clear by now that I believe lifestyle modifications should be our first line of defense in preventing coronary heart disease, I'm certainly not opposed to the use of medication when it's indicated. Sometimes we simply don't have the luxury of waiting for the beneficial effects of diet and exercise, and sometimes the best-designed diet and exercise just aren't enough. At such times, we need a more concentrated, immediate line of attack—and that's where medications come in. The medications in this chapter, whether taken alone or in combination, can help if your problem requires them.

I don't, however, subscribe to the one-drug-fits-all approach. Just as we've discussed in the lifestyle sections of this book, drug therapy is most likely to be successful if it is custom-fitted to the specific profile of an individual patient. And since these Advanced Metabolic Marker tests give us a much greater amount of information about the underlying conditions that are putting your heart at risk, they also facilitate a much more precise and personalized treatment strategy—and that includes the drugs you're on.

Obviously, the medications I'm discussing in this chapter are only available with a prescription, so this "Medication Prescription" shouldn't (and can't) be taken literally. These programs are merely intended as recommendations, to provide you with a launch pad for discussing various medication therapies with your doctor. I've included this chapter so that you can see what some of your medical options are: what the drugs are, how they do what they do, and some of the tips and tricks to reduce side effects and drug interactions that I've learned from my patients along the way. Remember, it is only appropriate to take a medication under the supervision of your physician.

You'll also find, in boxes throughout this chapter, information on other types of medications you may be taking that could have an effect on your heart. In the same way that our heart medications may affect other organs and parts of our bodies, the medications we take for other conditions may affect our heart. Some medications are very helpful, and others should go on a list of things to watch out for.

WHAT TO CONSIDER BEFORE YOU GO ON MEDICATION

So your doctor tells you that he'd like to see you on medication to correct some of your abnormal blood test numbers. That's good: It means that you're closing ranks and taking an aggressive approach toward cardiac prevention or treatment. But going on cardiac medication is a big step, and one that you won't want to take without doing due diligence.

So here are some issues that you'll want to cover with your physician before you begin any drug therapy.

- Should I get tested again?
- Do I have any other disorders that might be causing my abnormal results?
- What side effects should I be aware of?
- How long will I be on this drug?

Should I get tested again?

How reliable are these Advanced Metabolic Marker results? Can you trust the result to be conclusive? As I explained in chapter 5, there are some normal variations to be expected, either because you were having an "off" day, physiologically speaking, or because the lab was. Here is my general rule of thumb for answering those concerns.

If you're wildly high or wildly low, the variability matters less—even if the test is off, you're probably still high or low. But if you're borderline, I'd suggest getting tested again to ensure that you really do have one of these conditions. In other words, if your test results come back saying that your triglycerides are over 1,000 (when we like to see them around 70 and get alarmed at 140), then you need to be treated, no matter what. Even if it turns out that the test was off by 200 points one way or the other, you're still a good long way away from where you need to be. But if your test comes back and says that they're 170, which puts you 30 points above our alert value of 140, then you'd be wise to get another test before you decide to take medication to correct the problem, instead of first resorting to lifestyle modifications in order to close that smaller gap. You may have had a bowl of ice cream late the night before, so your triglycerides result of 170 milligrams per deciliter may not reflect your normal level.

The accuracy of your test results is of greater concern with this Prescription than it is with some of the lifestyle Prescriptions. If you have borderline readings that indicate you should be on a specific Exercise Plan, for instance, that's one thing. Borderline or no, starting an exercise program can only do you and your heart good! But if a borderline reading results in a lifelong drug therapy, that's another story. In my opinion, you want to be certain of a diagnosis before you begin medication, with all of its potential side effects and expense. So if your results are borderline, I'd suggest that you and your doctor seek further reassurance. In that case, taking the test again is a good idea. Again, review the material in chapter 5 about how to choose a reliable lab. If you are confident that the laboratory you used was reliable, then retest with that lab. (It is helpful to retest at the same lab, since there is always some variation between different laboratories, and that can confuse matters.)

Do I have any other disorders that might be causing my abnormal results?

It's good medicine to eliminate all other correctable disorders before prescribing medication, so your doctor will probably want to give you a thorough general checkup before putting you on medication.

Different parts of the body interact with one another, and conditions that affect other parts of the body may also result in abnormal marker or lipid numbers. Hypothyroidism, obstructive liver disease, pancreatic disease, and kidney disease can all contribute to abnormal numbers in your Advanced Metabolic Marker testing. For instance, a thyroid gland that's not working well can result in small LDL pattern B and elevated Lp(a), and other lipid disorders. Treating that underlying thyroid problem can cause those numbers to normalize. If this is the case, then thyroid hormone therapy is the logical next step, not lipid medications. That's why it's common to test thyroid function before prescribing lipid therapy.

Before you go on drug therapy, you and your doctor will want to make sure that you're treating a real metabolic condition and not the symptoms of another problem.

What side effects should I be aware of?

All drugs have side effects, though they may at times be so subtle that they go unnoticed. The drugs we'll primarily be talking about in this chapter are considered to be relatively safe, but it's important to note that all medications may have side effects, no matter how benign.

Before you begin a new medical treatment, ask your doctor what you should expect when you start taking the medication. Whenever you're prescribed a drug, you'll find that there's invariably a laundry list of scary-sounding side effects, and you may find the very existence of that list alarming. Don't worry, and please don't let that concern prevent you from educating yourself about them—you should know what the possible side effects are so you can promptly inform your doctor if you begin to experience them while you're on the drug.

The longer you're on a drug, the more likely it is that you'll experience side effects. Remember, you may tolerate a drug well for a year and then "suddenly" experience side effects. Since many of these drugs are prescribed with the assumption that the patient will be on them for the duration of his or her life, this is an important factor to consider. Ask your doctor how long he expects you to be on the drug. Good lifestyle habits can increase the chance that you'll be able to reduce the dose of the medication you take or stop taking it entirely (more on that later).

Although most of these drugs are very safe and are reported to have few side effects, idiosyncratic effects remain a possibility, and "new" side effects are linked to them all the time. For instance, a patient of mine who takes one of the statin drugs came in complaining of numbness in the toes of his left foot. He's an extremely experienced martial artist, and I made the assumption that he'd sustained nerve damage from kicking a punching bag over and over for 30 years and sent him away. Because there seemed to be a reasonable explanation for the symptom, I paid little attention to it. Then a short time later I read a new report stating that statin drugs had been linked to nerve damage. I immediately took him off the drugs, and the numbness improved.

> It's essential to check in with your physician regularly to make sure that you're not manifesting side effects. These regular checkups are especially important since you may not even know you're experiencing side effects without a blood test—sometimes the symptoms are silent until they're severe. If you're experiencing any of the side effects associated with the medication you're on, even if it's something trivial-seeming like a slight headache or an upset stomach and you think it's associated with the medication, let your physician know immediately.

It's important for you and your doctor to stay up to date on the emerging research about the drugs you're on, but there's another lesson here. This patient happened to be another physician, so he felt comfortable coming to me with what someone else might have dismissed as an unrelated complaint. But I've had patients who have suffered from side effects in silence because they didn't think to connect the discomfort they were encountering with the drug they were on. It's really important to let your doctor know immediately if you're experiencing any unexplained symptoms, so he or she can determine whether or not there's a connection.

In this chapter, we'll touch very generally on some of the side effects you might experience if you're taking these drugs. You should always have a complete and extensive conversation about side effects with your physician before you begin taking *any* medication. He or she will be aware of the drug's side-effect profile as determined by the Food and Drug Administration (FDA), the U.S. government agency responsible for approving new medications, and will be able to explain any possible side effects and adverse reactions in greater detail. You may also wish to discuss side-effect profiles with your pharmacist.

How long will I be on this drug?

This is an open-ended question that usually has to be left that way: Unless your doctor has a crystal ball, in most cases there's no way to predict how long you'll be on medication.

But that doesn't mean it shouldn't be asked. I'm always concerned about this because people do tend to stay on heart medication for a long period of time—if I diagnose a 50-year-old with high blood pressure and put him on a beta-blocker to bring his blood pressure down, he's going to be on that beta-blocker for a long, long time unless he finds some other way to control the problem.

Now, as we've already discussed, the longer you're on a medication, the more likely you are to experience side effects. And while we genuinely believe that these drugs are safe, many of the newer ones haven't been tested over a truly extended period of time. Many drug trials take place over 4 years or so, with a study population of 10,000. They can then say that they have 40,000 life years of information, but it's really only 4 years. We don't actually know how safe they are over the long haul. Plus, the cost of a lifelong drug therapy can really add up!

Medications to Watch Out For

Drug interactions are a serious business, and you should make certain that your doctor knows *all* of the drugs you take, *including* over-the-counter supplements and vitamins, before he or she prescribes any drug therapy.

Here are some of the ones that you might want to be aware of.

• Beta-blockers are a group of common prescription drugs used to control hypertension and other cardiovascular issues. However, many of them have also been shown to raise triglycerides and lower HDL levels. These drugs may also exacerbate the LDL pattern B, or small LDL, trait. If you're on a beta-blocker, your doctor should closely monitor your lipid levels and advise you on a lipid-controlling therapy if necessary. If you're taking a beta-blocker for blood-pressure control and your triglycerides are elevated or your HDL-C is low, you and your doctor may want to consider switching you to a different type of blood pressure medication to control the problem before starting a second drug to treat the triglycerides and HDL.

• Many patients don't think of their psychopharmacological drugs—their antidepressants or their anxiety medication—in the same way that they think of the drugs they take for their physical health and often leave them off the list they give their doctor. These are drugs like all other drugs and should be included. Tricyclic antidepressants have an impact on lipid metabolism, for instance.

• Birth control pills contain estrogen and can raise triglycerides if you're already susceptible to elevated levels. When someone's triglycerides are dangerously high, one option is always to take them off the birth control pills.

• Some antiepilepsy drugs can raise homocysteine levels.

So you'll want to have a conversation to find out what your doctor has in mind. Ask your doctor if it's realistic to aim toward backing off medication entirely in the future, if your lifestyle changes and improved blood work permit.

THE ARGUMENT FOR COMBINATION THERAPIES

As you'll see, many of the medication therapies I'm discussing in this chapter are **combination therapies**, which is to say that they combine one or more drugs to achieve the desired effect.

There are a number of reasons why I like using these combination therapies. First of all, if you're using two different drugs, then you can often use a lower dose of each drug. When you're on lower doses of each drug, you're less likely to experience side effects from either of them.

No One Drug Fits All

But the other side of my passion for these combination therapies is that I believe it's the best way to treat the *whole* patient. Our war against LDL cholesterol as the major villain of the coronary heart disease story has led us down a dangerous path. Since the statin drugs are the easiest and most effective way to lower LDL cholesterol, it seems like everyone's on a statin.

There's no denying how effective these drugs are, but they're primarily effective at lowering LDL cholesterol and have much less of an impact on triglycerides and HDLs. When we focus exclusively on this LDL cholesterol issue, we neglect other, very real conditions that may be putting you at risk for coronary heart disease—in some cases, even more risk than LDL alone!

Once you look at the Medication Prescription Key for this chapter, you'll see I'm certainly not shying away from "prescribing" statins. These drugs are very, very good at lowering the mass of atherogenic particles that includes LDLs. So if your only problem is high LDL-C, then they're the only therapy you may need to pursue (although even in this case, I like to combine them with a low dose of another drug). In many cases, people have other, serious metabolic issues as well as high LDL-C, and they need to look elsewhere for a solution. Statins do very little for your HDL, or your Lp(a), and although they do lower the overall mass of LDL, they don't do anything to convert you from the dangerous LDL pattern B to the less harmful LDL pattern A. As we've learned, these are not things we can afford to ignore.

How, then, can we avoid this one-drug-fits-all path? There are a number of really good, powerful, time-tested drugs that can be used in combination with the statins and *do* correct these other underlying metabolic issues. Niacin, for instance, can change your LDL pattern B to LDL pattern A, and it can increase your HDL2b and lower your Lp(a). Niacin is less effective at lowering LDL-C, an area where the statin drugs excel. So the niacin-statin combination is a terrific one if you have high LDL-C and apo B, as well as one of these other metabolic issues, like low HDL2b, high triglycerides, LDL pattern B, or high Lp(a). And other combinations are possible as well. The first study to show that heart disease regression was possible was Dr. David Blankenhorn's Cholesterol Lowering and Atherosclerosis Study (CLAS), which used a resin plus niacin.

THE BEST COMBINATION THERAPY OF ALL: MEDICATION *AND* LIFESTYLE MODIFICATIONS

In my experience, the combination therapy with the best results takes place when the right medication is combined with the right lifestyle modification.

I really do encourage you to use all four components of the Prescriptions in this book in concert, giving as much weight to the lifestyle elements as you do to this chapter on medication. If your lifestyle is less than optimal, I strongly recommend that you make every effort to begin the programs assigned to you in this book and maintain those necessary lifestyle changes *as well* as taking the drugs your doctor prescribes. No magic pill can make up for a pack-a-day cigarette habit, and a great diet and exercise program stands a good chance of reducing the dose of the drug you need. The lower the dose, the less expensive it will be, and the less likely you are to experience side effects.

And in some cases, the lifestyle changes you make may have a profound enough effect that you'll eventually be able to back away from the medication entirely! If your doctor prescribes medication, I recommend that you follow that therapy path—as well as making lifestyle changes—for approximately 3 to 4 months, and then have your blood work redone to see if your numbers have improved. If they have, you and your doctor may eventually want to talk about lowering the dose or backing off medication completely. Pound for pound, the medications often work more effectively when you also improve lifestyle issues.

You may even want to make a verbal agreement with your doctor to take

Timing Tip

Throughout this chapter, you'll find these Timing Tip boxes, with advice on the best time to take your medications.

Although taking your medications at certain times of day *can* help you maximize their effectiveness, these Timing Tips are merely suggestions.

When's the absolute best time to take your medication? The real answer to this question, of course, is: **whenever you're most likely to remember to take it**. A fancy dosing schedule does no one any good if you're just going to miss your pill every day because you're "supposed" to take it at a time that's inconvenient for you. So if you can accommodate these timing suggestions into your daily life easily, please do so. But if you're most likely to remember to take your pill when you're having your orange juice in the morning or before you brush your teeth at night, then those are the best times to take it.

another look at your dosage if you're able to improve your physiology through exercise and diet—by losing 15 pounds, for instance, or converting yourself from LDL pattern B to LDL pattern A through diet and daily exercise.

The Other Benefits of Medication

Your doctor may have other reasons for wanting you to stay on medication, though. Many of these drugs have what are called pleiotropic effects—in other words, they have positive effects above and beyond the reason you're taking them, and your doctor may feel that you're reaping some other benefits from continuing with them. I've included some of the widely accepted pleiotropic effects in our discussion of these drugs. Again, the decision to continue with medication is something that you'll want to discuss in detail with your physician.

FINDING YOUR MEDICATION PRESCRIPTION

As with the Nutrition, Exercise, and Supplement components of this program, you'll use the Prescription Key on page 251 to help you locate the individualized Medication Plan that has been calibrated to meet the needs of your particular cardiac profile. All you'll need to do is match the results of your own tests against the Prescription Key to find the plan that is right for you.

The first plan, the **Cholesterol Knockout Plan**, is designed to combat our old enemy, high LDL cholesterol (the "bad" cholesterol) and its partner in crime, high apo B—and I'll show you how it puts LDL pattern B in its crosshairs as well. The next plan, the **Heavyweight Plan**, uses our most powerful weapons to help people struggling with a number of hard-to-fight issues, including LDL pattern B, high Lp(a), low HDL2b (and its own partner in crime, elevated triglycerides). And the final plan, the **One-Two Punch Plan**, comprises combination therapies: statins plus either niacin or fibrates, which will launch an intensive, multipronged attack on a combination of disorders.

Note: My goal in this chapter is to show you how our knowledge of these additional markers can help doctors in determining the right therapy for you and to show you the thinking behind the decision to take one medication path over another. You'll also find tips and tricks to help you cope with some of the common side effects caused by these medications. Since these medications are available only by prescription and should in no case be taken except under medical supervision, this is merely intended to be an exploration of your options. It is certainly not meant to supplant your relationship with your doctor, but to enable you to participate in your care in an active and informed way.

Using the Prescription Key

Directly below the Medication Prescription Key on the opposite page you'll see a list of four markers labeled "My Medication Markers." These will determine which individualized Medication Plan is the right fit for your cardiac profile.

Refer back to your Quick Reference Chart on page 91 to help you to fill in a "yes" or "no" in the space provided beside each Medication Marker. (Let's do an example together: Paul has tested "abnormal" on LDL pattern B and HDL2b, but "normal" on Lp(a) and apo B. So his column would read "Yes," "Yes," "No," "No.")

Once you have your list of yeses and no's, just look up at the Key and find the column that duplicates your pattern. (Remember, read down the columns, from top to bottom, until you find your exact match.)

The Medication Prescription Key

Medication Marker															
LDL pattern B	Yes	Yes	Yes	Yes	Yes	Yes	Yes	Yes	Yes	No	No	No	No	No	No
HDL2b	No	Yes	No	No	No	No	No	Yes	Yes	No	No	No	Yes	Yes	No
Lp(a)	No	No	Yes	Yes	No	Yes	Yes	Yes	Yes	No	Yes	No	Yes	No	Yes
Apo B	No	No	Yes	Yes	Yes	Yes	Yes	Yes	Yes	Yes	No	Yes	No	No	No
Medication Plan #:	2	2	2	2	3	3	3	3	3	1	N/A	3	2	2	2

Medication Plan #1: THE CHOLESTEROL KNOCKOUT PLAN
Medication Plan #2: THE HEAVYWEIGHT PLAN
Medication Plan #3: THE ONE-TWO PUNCH PLAN

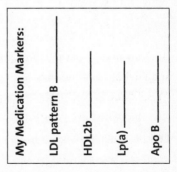

My Medication Markers:

LDL pattern B _____

HDL2b _____

Lp(a) _____

Apo B _____

At the base of the column that matches your own results, you'll find the number that identifies *your* plan! (Paul would find the plan that matches *his* pattern in the second column from the left. Since the number at the base of the column is 2, he should proceed to the second Medication Plan, the Heavyweight Plan.)

So refer back to your Quick Reference Chart on page 91, and let's get started.

Note: If you haven't taken the Advanced Metabolic Marker tests or if you're still waiting for your results, don't worry. Even though we can't direct you to a plan, you can still gain plenty of information by reading through them. In my practice I won't prescribe medications for my patients before carefully analyzing their Advanced Metabolic Marker tests: Without those results I can't deliver really top-of-the-line, patient-specific care. I can't in good faith treat my patients without this additional knowledge, and I can't make suggestions to you and your physician here about medications unless you know the status of your own advanced markers.

That said, even without the testing, there's plenty for you to do in order to begin your journey down the road to lifelong heart health. Be sure to follow the Nutrition and Exercise Prescriptions that have been assigned to you! If you decide to get tested in the future, then you'll be able to insert your numbers into the Prescription Key and find out which plan is right for you.

So let's move on to our individualized Medication Prescriptions!

MEDICATION PLAN #1
THE CHOLESTEROL KNOCKOUT PLAN

This first Medication Plan stands as proof that I'm not ignoring good old cholesterol, despite my enthusiasm for these new Advanced Metabolic Markers.

Approximately half of all middle-aged men have high cholesterol, and it remains one of the classic risk factors for coronary artery disease. In fact, LDL, particularly when it becomes oxidized, is one of the leading scoundrels in the war we're waging against coronary heart disease. When I see high LDL cholesterol, I treat it, and the drugs we use with this plan, the statins, the resin drugs, and a new drug called ezetimibe (either alone or in combination with one another), are among the best ways to control this pervasive problem.

But what about all our fancy new tests, you might be asking. Haven't we left cholesterol behind? On the contrary, you'll see that our Advanced Metabolic Marker tests actually provide us with *further* reasons to stay on top of this cholesterol issue.

Who Should Use This Medication Plan?

- People with elevated apo B
- People with elevated LDL-C

People with Elevated Apo B and LDL-C

We can't really separate apo B from LDL cholesterol, because when we talk about "oxidized LDL," we're actually talking about oxidized apo B.

To refresh your memory, apo B is the protein that hangs off the LDL molecule, and it's prone to dangerous oxidization. Each LDL has one, and only one, apo B attached to it, so determining the amount of apo B gives you a very accurate measure of the number of these dangerous particles circulating in your bloodstream.

When apo B becomes oxidized, it becomes very, very yummy-looking to the macrophages, which are white blood cells designed to clean up the artery walls. So they gobble up tons of this LDL with the attractive-looking oxidized apo B, and they eventually become obese, turning into what we call foam cells because their insides are filled with fat that looks like foam. As these foam cells get bigger and bigger, they threaten the stability of the plaque in the artery, and when they rupture, it can cause a cardiac event.

So when you have elevated apo B, it means that you have a lot of these particles that are prone to oxidation, and that's a process we want to stop before it starts. Lowering apo B by reducing the amount of the LDL it hangs out on is one good way to do that.

Lowering Cholesterol and LDL Pattern B

Our Cholesterol Knockout Plan will also help people with LDL pattern B. Now, you may notice that LDL pattern B people are directed to other Medication Plans. That's simply because there are better drugs to convert people from LDL pattern B to LDL pattern A. The statin and resin drugs and ezetimibe lower the *number* of LDLs in your system—they don't change the subclass distribution. In other words, they lower your overall LDL count, but they won't take you from the perilous LDL pattern B to the safer LDL pattern A. That doesn't mean that lowering LDL cholesterol doesn't make a significant difference in this LDL pattern B issue.

How does it work? Let's say you have 200 LDLs—100 of them are the large, less-atherogenic particles, and the other 100 are the dangerous small LDLs. If you can reduce your overall LDLs by half, that will definitely make a difference: The 50 small LDLs that you're left with after treatment is a much better scenario than the 100 you started out with. Other drugs can change the *distribution* of your LDLs. Niacin, for instance, can help you to convert those 50 remaining small LDLs into larger, less dangerous particles. In fact, that's the logic behind many of the combination therapies you'll find in these Medication Plans. A niacin-statin combination, for instance, is the ideal one-two punch: You use the statins or resins to reduce the overall LDLs and then niacin or a fibrate to move what's left into the less-atherogenic category. But, of course, simply reducing the *number* of the small LDLs you have in circulation is an absolute asset and will have a beneficial result on your heart health.

The three major categories of drugs that we use to treat high LDL-C and elevated apo B are the statins, the resins, and ezetimibe. Let's explore each in greater detail.

STATINS

The statin drugs have completely revolutionized the blood-cholesterol treatment industry. Prior to their appearance, the main drugs used to reduce LDL-C were the bile acid–binding resins (and more on them in a minute), which required that you mix a sandy material into a liquid and drink it a number of times a day. After that, a single pill that only needed to be taken once a day was a real gift to those who required LDL-C reduction. The bile acid–binding resins have gotten *much easier* to take, but the statins have really taken off.

Common Names

Some of the most common statin names are atorvastatin (marketed as Lipitor), fluvastatin (Lescol), lovastatin (Mevacor), pravastatin (Pravachol), and simvastatin (Zocor). This is one of the fastest-developing drug markets, so new products appear regularly.

What They Do

The statin drugs are derived from an Asian fungus that has been used to combat coronary heart disease for thousands of years and one that is still found in Asian herbal treatments. The statins are astonishingly effective at lowering the mass of LDL, and they're very easy to take, which explains their tremendous popularity. They've been shown to reduce LDL cholesterol significantly—between 30 and 50 percent. They may also raise HDL slightly (between 5 and 15 percent) and lower triglycerides (between 7 and 30 percent), but they're primarily used to lower LDL-C.

How They Work

Statins slow the liver's production of cholesterol and increase the liver's ability to remove LDL from the bloodstream. The drugs block the activity of an enzyme called HMG-CoA reductase, which helps your liver to make cholesterol (for this reason, the statin drugs are also called HMG-CoA reductase inhibitors).

As you'll remember, there are special receptors in the liver that recognize and grab LDL when the body needs cholesterol. When your liver makes less cholesterol (because the statin is inhibiting it from doing so), it interprets that cholesterol deficit as a *need* for cholesterol, so it increases the LDL receptors in the liver in order to pull more cholesterol from the blood. The more LDL receptors you have, the more efficiently the liver is pulling LDL from the bloodstream. That naturally lowers the blood level of LDL-C.

Side Effects

In general, the statins are fairly well-tolerated. There are, however, some side effects associated with them.

Gastrointestinal Distress

There's a low instance of gastrointestinal side effects, including constipation and gas, and there have also been some reports of sleep disturbances associated with the statin drugs, but these are relatively uncommon.

Increase in Liver Function

Potentially more serious side effects include an increase in liver function. If tests show only slightly elevated function, there is little practical significance, but really high levels may reflect a drug-induced liver dysfunction. Sometimes there are no associated symptoms with liver dysfunction, so it's essential that you see your physician every 6 months for a blood test when you're on these drugs. If a blood sample shows that your liver functions are increased, and there's no other reason for them to be elevated—because you've been drinking heavily, for instance, or you've been sick—then he may test you again in a week to confirm that they're still elevated. If those levels are high enough, he'll adjust the medication accordingly.

If you're on these drugs and suddenly find yourself feeling nauseated or with the symptoms of a bad flu, then you should call your doctor's office immediately. If your liver function is significantly elevated—three times the upper limit of normal—your doctor will probably assume the drug is implicated and stop it immediately. He'll check the levels again in a week or so and may restart the drug if your levels are normal. You'll find out fast if the drug caused the elevation or if you actually had the flu.

Muscle Inflammation

Another potentially serious side effect with the statins is the possibility of muscle inflammation, which manifests itself in muscle pain or discomfort. It feels like you've run a marathon or like the kind of achiness you feel when you're coming down with the flu—especially if you squeeze the belly of the

CHECK IN REGULARLY WITH YOUR DOCTOR

I want to emphasize the tremendous importance of routine safety evaluations. You must check in with your physician at regularly scheduled intervals when you're taking medication. Just because you tolerate a drug very well at the beginning of the therapy doesn't mean that you don't need to be monitored going forward. Don't miss your checkups!

muscle. This condition, called myositis, is certainly uncomfortable and can be very serious if it leads to muscle breakdown, which can result in protein deposits in the kidneys—and kidney failure or even death. While this reaction is really very rare, if it occurs it can be quite serious, so if you think you have symptoms of myositis while on these medications, call your physician.

Dehydration

One thing that does tend to affect people on statins is dehydration. When you aren't diligent about replacing your fluids, you get dehydrated. The amount of water in your blood goes down, and since you have less water, there's automatically a higher concentration of the drug in your bloodstream, which can increase the side effects of the drug you're on. If you're on a statin, that can lead to this muscle inflammation we've talked about.

So if you're on a statin, make sure to drink lots of water, especially when you're exercising—and that's good advice for everyone, medicated or not.

Contraindications

In some cases, the statins may not be the right drug for you, either because of other medical conditions you might have—or what you like to drink with your breakfast!

Timing Tip

Take your statin drug at night. The body makes more cholesterol at night and in the early morning hours, so it is often more effective at blocking production if you take it with your evening meal or at bedtime.

Grapefruit Juice

Interestingly, ordinary grapefruit juice may seriously interfere with your body's metabolism of statin drugs. Your body clears these drugs from your system through a natural process that requires an enzyme. Grapefruit juice interferes with that enzyme, blocking the body's ability to clear statins from the bloodstream, and this can contribute to the muscle inflammation we discussed previously. This particular side effect happens less frequently with the newer drugs.

Kidney and Liver Disease

Muscle inflammation, or myositis, tends to be worse in people with other diseases—kidney disease, existing liver disease, or those taking drugs that have an adverse effect on the liver. In fact, this side effect was first discovered in heart transplant patients who were taking an immunosuppressant called cyclosporine, which reduces the chance that the body will reject the new organ. People with poorly working kidneys can also get into trouble with the statins because the blood level of the drug is higher than it would be if the kidneys were working normally. So statin drugs are often contraindicated for people with preexisting liver and kidney conditions and people who are taking drugs that tax these organs.

> **Cardiac medications are designed to treat coronary heart disease, but their side effects aren't necessarily limited to your heart! Your physician must always have a complete medical history on you and a current picture of your medical and drug profile before he or she can safely prescribe a drug. Don't leave anything out, no matter how minor or unrelated it might seem.**

Other Benefits

Statins are terrific at lowering LDL cholesterol, and that's primarily what we use them for, but they're reported to have other benefits as well. They're said to improve vasoreactivity—to relax the arteries, making them less prone to spasm. They're also reported to lower hs-CRP, and thus may play some role in protecting the heart with an anti-inflammatory effect. Unlike some of the other cholesterol-lowering drugs, there's the hint that there may be fewer cancer events with the statins than in people on other drugs: There's slim evidence (from studies that weren't designed to explore this issue) that in the test tube, the statins may decrease cell reproduction in certain cell lines that have been linked to cancer.

BILE ACID–BINDING RESINS (RESINS)

So with drugs as good at lowering LDL as the statins, who could ask for anything more?

In this case, our alternative to lower your LDL-C and apo B are the bile acid binders, or resin drugs (sometimes also called bile acid sequestrants). I love using these resins because they're extremely safe medicines—they've been around for a long time and there are no really serious recorded side effects as a result of long-term use. One of the reasons for this is that they never actually enter your bloodstream; they stay in the intestines, do their job, and then you eliminate them with other waste when you go to the bathroom.

This is why they're such a good alternative to the statins. Sometimes I do encounter patients who have had negative reactions to the statin drugs. Sometimes my patients are simply concerned—they know the statin drugs are relatively new, and they know that they're likely to be on the drugs for a good long time, so they're worried that side effects will crop up. And often the decision is my own. If I had a young patient who was going to need to be on LDL-lowering medication for a long time, I might start with a resin because they're really safe drugs. When we're talking about someone who's looking at spending the next 50 years on drug therapy, long-term safety is my first priority.

As you'll see, these two categories of drugs aren't mutually exclusive—they're also very effective in combination with one another. So your physician may want to mix and match, according to your specific needs.

These resin drugs originally fell out of favor because they can have some gastrointestinal side effects and because they were quite inconvenient to take. They used to come exclusively in a powder form, which you had to mix into water and drink a number of times a day, a process that someone famously compared to drinking sand. Obviously, this was unpleasant compared to the statins, which are once-a-day pills. But there's now a resin in pill form, which makes it much more user-friendly, and I use these drugs whenever they're appropriate.

Common Names
Some of the most common resin names are cholestyramine (Questran), colestipol hydrochloride (Colestid), and colesevelam (WelChol).

What They Do
The resins lower LDL cholesterol. They have little or no effect on HDL-C, and in some cases, they can cause triglycerides to increase.

How They Work
Bile is broken-down cholesterol—a cholesterol building block, if you will. After you eat, your gallbladder squirts bile into the intestines to help dissolve fat. When the bile has done its job, it's reabsorbed into the intestines and goes back to the gallbladder.

These bile acid–binding drugs don't allow that reabsorption process; they bind to the bile so that it's eliminated with the other waste in your stool. Of course, your body perceives this shortage of bile as a cholesterol deficit, so it up-regulates, or increases the production of, these special receptors that recognize and suck up LDL from the bloodstream when the body needs cholesterol. More LDL receptors means that they can pull more LDL cholesterol

Timing Tip
The ideal time to take the resin drugs is a half hour before dinner (or your largest meal of the day). By the time the food reaches your intestine, the drug is already in an ideal position to go to work.

Medication Tip

Increasing your fiber intake and drinking lots of water can help with some of the gastrointestinal discomfort that may accompany resin therapy.

from your bloodstream, and that causes the amount of LDL-C in your bloodstream to go down.

Side Effects

Although the bile acid binders are very safe over the long term, they can have some uncomfortable short-term side effects.

Gastrointestinal Distress

The primary side effects of these bile acid binders are gastrointestinal: constipation, bloating, and gas. This is definitely dose related—these side effects are less often experienced by people on low doses of the resins. We've also discovered in the clinic that mixing a teaspoon of psyllium (Metamucil) into the dose significantly reduces the discomfort, as does a tablespoon of mineral oil a day. Drinking lots of water always helps.

Binding Other Medications

Another potential problem with the resins is that they can bind other things—not just bile—in your bloodstream. Those things include other medications, like thyroid replacement hormones and antibiotics, and folic acid. If the resins bind with medication, the medication won't get absorbed, and if they bind with folic acid, your homocysteine may go up. A solution that works very well is simply to take the bile acid binder at a different time of day than you take your other medications.

Timing Tip

Resins may also bind with your other medications, which will prevent them from being absorbed. Take them at different times of the day—your other meds in the morning and your bile acid binder at night—and you should be able to avoid a problem.

Contraindications

As terrific as these drugs are, they're not the right medication for everyone.

High Triglycerides

The resin drugs can raise your triglycerides, so they're contraindicated if your triglycerides are already high. This is a case where we'd use a statin drug instead to control your LDL issue or a resin plus niacin.

Serious Gastrointestinal Problems

Since the resins can cause gastrointestinal distress, if you have serious gastrointestinal problems, like chronic constipation, diverticulitis, or ulcerative colitis, you and your doctor will probably want to discuss other medication options, like the statins, which are less irritating to this part of the body.

Other Potential Benefits

There are no pleiotropic effects to be had from the resin drugs, as far as we know.

THE STATIN-RESIN COMBINATION

If the intent of the therapy is to lower cholesterol, then I like to use a combination of a low-dose statin and a low-dose resin. You can see up to a 50 percent reduction in LDL cholesterol, and with a reduced risk of side effects and overall systemic risk than from a single-drug therapy. I'm a fan of multiple-drug therapies for precisely this reason: You can use much lower doses of the individual drugs, which lowers the risk of side effects—with the same results. It can even be *more* effective than single doses of either drug, since these drugs amplify each other's effects.

The statin-resin combination is time honored and has been used in a number of influential studies sponsored by the National Institutes of Health, including the Familial Atherosclerosis Treatment Study (FATS) and the Stan-

OTHER MEDICATIONS THAT MAY HELP YOUR HEART: HORMONE THERAPY

When a woman goes through menopause, the level of the hormone estrogen drops in her system. Hormone therapy (HT) is a system of drugs that replaces lowered estrogen and progesterone. HT has always been controversial: Many women (and many physicians) feel that menopause isn't a disease and shouldn't require extensive drug therapy.

One of the strongest arguments made in favor of HT has been the associated health benefit. As we know, the presence of estrogen appears to protect women from many cardiovascular ills, and when the body stops producing the hormone in the same quantities, those protective benefits are lost. Replacing the hormone should then reinstate the benefits.

Recently, several major long-term studies of women on hormone therapy have been reported. One was stopped early because of elevated cancer rates, and that has made estrogen therapy all the more controversial. Another study in postmenopausal women with coronary heart disease showed no heart disease reduction in the group of women who took HT—in fact, there was a slight increase in adverse cardiac events in the first year of starting HT. But in that same study, 25 percent of the women with elevated Lp(a) showed a significant reduction in heart events attributed to the HT's effect on lowering Lp(a).

This is a good example of the necessity for individualized, personalized patient care—and for knowing what your Lp(a) level is!

Knowing whether or not you're predominantly LDL pattern B can also factor into a decision about HT. In one study, LDL pattern B women on HT lowered their LDL 15 percent—while LDL pattern As on HT only dropped 4.6 percent. The "good" HDL rose 14 percent in the LDL pattern B women, but only 8 percent in the LDL pattern As. We think that estrogen suppresses the genes that cause coronary heart disease in LDL pattern B women, and that when menopause sets in, they lose the benefits of estrogen. This is another area where our Advanced Metabolic Marker testing really helps us when we're deciding on treatment.

There are many factors to consider before recommending that a patient pursue a therapy, especially one with risk factors. But the benefit of any treatment should always outweigh its risks.

ford Coronary Risk Intervention Project (SCRIP), which showed definite evidence of arteriographic improvement.

EZETIMIBE

Ezetimibe is a new medication to lower cholesterol. When used by itself, it lowers LDL-C about 18 percent but in combination with one of the statins, it can lower LDL-C 50 to 60 percent.

Common Name
This drug is also called Zetia.

How It Works
Ezetimibe works by blocking cholesterol absorption through the intestines. This is essentially the same thing that the resin drugs do, but the mechanism is a little different. Ultimately though, like the resins, ezetimibe results in a reduction in the intestinal cholesterol delivery to the liver—and the end result is lower LDL-C.

Side Effects
This drug seems to be very well-tolerated. Some patients have reported the following side effects.

Gastrointestinal Distress
Some patients have complained of diarrhea and stomach pain as a result of this drug.

Fatigue
People have also noticed an increased feeling of fatigue when on this medication.

Myositis
The muscle inflammation described in the statin section may occur with this drug when it is taken in combination with the statin drugs.

MEDICATION PLAN #1:
THE CHOLESTEROL KNOCKOUT PLAN

Statin, Resin, Statin + Resin, Ezetimibe, or Ezetimibe + Statin
    It is only appropriate to take medication under the supervision of a physician.

Contraindications
People with Gastrointestinal Disease
People who already experience gastrointestinal difficulty, such as a history of ulcerative colitis or peptic ulcers, will want to avoid this drug and its potential side effects.

People with Liver Disease
People with liver disease should not take this medication, especially in combination with the statin drugs.

Other Benefits
We are not yet aware of any pleiotropic effects to be had from this drug.

MEDICATION PLAN #2
THE HEAVYWEIGHT PLAN

In this plan, we use niacin and fibrates, two of the classic cardiac heavyweights. These two types of drugs cross swords against the unholy trinity of coronary heart disease: They lower triglycerides, boost the protective HDL, and reduce small LDL.

Who Should Use This Medication Plan?

- People with elevated triglycerides
- People with low HDL2b
- People with LDL pattern B
- People with high Lp(a)

These are both drugs that have been around for a long time, and I feel that they're relatively safe, so I like using them.

People with Elevated Triglycerides

Both niacin and fibrates lower triglycerides. But triglycerides aren't an advanced marker, and they're certainly not one of our Medication Markers—so why are they included here?

First of all, high triglycerides are an independent marker for coronary heart disease, so it's always a good idea to lower them if they're high. But this triglyceride issue is central to a number of other metabolic interactions.

Very low-density lipoproteins (VLDLs) are essentially big bubbles that carry a lot of triglycerides. As you'll remember from the Exercise Prescription, the enzyme lipoprotein lipase (LPL) brushes up against these VLDLs and chews up the triglycerides inside the bubble. During that process, surface components break off and are released into the bloodstream. Those surface proteins are building blocks available for HDL. So when you lower your triglycerides, you're making more building blocks for the creation of HDL. And the fewer triglycerides you have, the fewer VLDLs and intermediate-density lipoproteins (IDLs) you'll have. These particles are much more susceptible to harmful oxidation, so lowering the number of them is another step in the right direction.

People with Low HDL2b

Your body has its own built-in arterial defense system in the form of the "good" HDL, which takes cholesterol out of the arterial walls and returns it to the liver for recycling. And this good cholesterol also carries a potent natural antioxidant, so it confers some protective benefits against the ravages of oxidation as well. But this natural fortification—one of your best defenses against coronary heart disease—is constantly under attack. Two of our best sandbags to shore up your body's natural defenses are these two drugs: niacin and the fibrates.

As we'll see, niacin and the fibrates raise HDL using two different mechanisms. First of all, they both help to lower triglycerides, which releases more of those building blocks into the bloodstream. The fibrates actually instruct the genes to make more of the building blocks for HDL, and niacin prevents HDL from degrading, so they both contribute to increased amounts of this important lipoprotein.

People with LDL Pattern B

We don't actually know the exact mechanism by which niacin helps to convert people from pattern B to pattern A. What we do know is that it's the best drug for this particular purpose in existence. The fibrates also do this, but slightly less effectively, mostly because we can increase the dose of niacin, while the fibrate dose is fixed.

People with High Lp(a)

Most of the Advanced Metabolic Markers we've discussed have clear treatment paths: lose weight, cut the fat in your diet, take this pill. And thankfully, most of them are very responsive to the right kind of treatment.

The real holdout is unfortunately one of the most serious: lipoprotein (a), which can raise your risk of coronary heart dease by 300 percent. Lp(a) is a kind of LDL with an abnormal protein attached to it, and it carries its own set of dangers, including inflammation and encouraging the growth of smooth muscle tissue, but it's also *extremely* prone to the damaging oxidation process.

But unlike so many of these other markers, Lp(a) doesn't care if you lose 10 pounds or learn to kickbox. It doesn't respond to the snazziest new drugs on the market. The two things it seems to respond to are hormone therapy (HT) and niacin. HT is a controversial solution and one that only applies to women—which leaves us with niacin as the best weapon against this abnormal protein.

NIACIN (NICOTINIC ACID)

This may surprise you, but nicotinic acid, or niacin, is actually just a B vitamin. It's an over-the-counter supplement, in fact. We'll discuss supplements

Medication Tip

When I say niacin, I mean nicotinic acid. *Niacinamide* is another chemical compound that also goes under the name niacin—but it has no lipid-cardiac benefits. The two should not be confused.

in greater detail in the next chapter, but since we're talking about some very high dosages here, ones that you absolutely shouldn't take unless you're under a doctor's supervision, I've included niacin with the prescription drugs.

I believe very strongly in this therapy: It's inexpensive, it's been used to treat lipid disorders for decades, it's been the subject of many successful studies that demonstrate improved heart disease outcomes, and it's relatively safe. Although it hasn't been monitored by the U.S. Food and Drug Administration for very long, there's lots of data on it, and the anecdotal evidence of the doctors that use it is overwhelmingly positive. So I feel very confident using this drug over an extended period of time.

Common Names

These drugs are also called nicotinic acid, Niaspan, and Slo Niacin.

What It Does

Niacin has been shown to consistently lower total cholesterol, LDL cholesterol (by 15 to 20 percent), and triglycerides (by 10 to 40 percent) while raising HDL (by 15 to 40 percent). In other words, it improves the ratio of good to bad cholesterols. The effect of niacin is dose related: The more you take, the greater the effect. This is a good thing because it allows your physician to titrate, or gradually increase, the dose of the drug to achieve the desired effect. It can also reduce small LDL and Lp(a).

LDL pattern B people tend to respond better to niacin than LDL pattern As. It's one of the best drugs to drive reverse cholesterol transport and can result in quite substantial increases in the good HDL2b. It has been demonstrated that a niacin therapy reduces the risk of a second heart attack and can

PRESCRIPTION VERSUS
OVER-THE-COUNTER NIACIN

There are two different kinds of niacin on the market: regular immediate-release niacin and time-release niacin, which is a prescription drug marketed under the name Niaspan. Each has its pros and cons. The immediate release is a little higher maintenance. It needs to be taken two to three times a day, and because the niacin is released immediately, side effects tend to be more pronounced.

Niaspan has gone through a full round of U.S. Food and Drug Administration (FDA) testing and has been approved for use. It releases slowly into the bloodstream, so that there's less instance of the side effects usually associated with this drug. You take a single dose at bedtime, which means that it's easier to remember to take it. Some patients feel comforted by the fact that it's gone through the FDA approval process as well. This process gathers accurate data on side effects and the kind of lipid response you can realistically expect. The FDA also monitors the production of Niaspan in the factory, so I feel comfortable that the production quality control is consistently good.

The biggest drawback with Niaspan is that you're limited to the FDA's dose limit, which is 2,000 milligrams a day, a relatively low dose. It's been known for quite some time that when used in high doses, niacin can cause elevated liver function and may cause a form of chemical hepatitis in doses higher than the standard dosage that most doctors would recommend. Still, to be on the safe side, the FDA set the maximum daily dose at 2,000 milligrams. This works out fine because now we often use niacin in combination with other lipid-lowering medications, like the resins and the statins.

If you're going with over-the-counter niacin, I believe it is worth the additional expense to go with the brands that are known to be reputable and reliable. There's no regulatory agency overseeing the quality of non-prescription drugs. So there can be a real problem getting consistency in the strength and the purity of the drug, especially if you're switching between brands. In my experience, a Squibb subsidiary called Apothecon and another company called Twinlab are two companies that make over-the-counter niacin and have good quality control.

reduce the rate of coronary heart disease buildup in the coronary arteries as well as actually regressing the disease in some people.

How It Works

Niacin effectively confronts a number of different and equally important issues. Niacin decreases liver production of LDL and converts your existing LDL into a less destructive form. It also protects HDL by slowing the rate at which it degrades. This keeps it around longer, which results in much higher amounts of HDL-C and HDL2b. Although it's not its primary role, niacin may also increase the activity of the enzyme lipoprotein lipase, which lowers triglycerides and increases the good HDL. And it may decrease the activity of LPL's evil twin hepatic lipase, which promotes the expression of the small LDL trait.

Side Effects

The most common side effects of niacin include skin flushing, hot flashes, nausea, gas, and gastrointestinal distress. These aren't serious in most cases, but they can be uncomfortable. Although very few people do experience serious side effects from niacin, there are some that you should be aware of, and I'd like to talk about those first.

Raised Uric Acid Levels

Niacin may sometimes raise uric acid levels in the bloodstream of some (but not all) people. When uric acid levels get high enough, they can cause gout attacks. Gout is a genetic disease, triggered when uric acid crystals get into a joint. It's excruciatingly painful, but it won't kill you. Before we put a patient on niacin, we check his uric acid levels. If they're high or if he has a history of gout, we'll use a drug called allopurinol to help keep uric acid levels down. If you don't have a genetic potential for gout, it is highly unlikely that niacin will cause this problem.

Irregular Heartbeat

Another potential adverse effect of niacin is a slightly higher incidence of atrial fibrillation. The heartbeat normally starts in the small upper chambers of the heart and moves on to the large lower chamber. Atrial fibrillation is a shaking in the upper chamber. If the upper chamber shakes, the lower chambers start beating faster as well, which is not a good thing and may contribute to irregular heartbeat. Ironically, if you're in chronic atrial fibrillation, we just go ahead and treat you with niacin. It's when you're going in and out of atrial fibrillation that you can get a blood clot, which can then break off during a regular contraction and cause a brain infarct or pulmonary embolism. This is generally a problem found in people who already have coronary heart disease. If you're going in and out of atrial fibrillation, I would not recommend niacin for you.

Liver Inflammation

There's also the risk of liver inflammation when you take niacin at extremely high doses. Normally, such inflammation occurs only at much higher doses than the ones used to improve your cardiac profile, but if you're on a high dose of niacin, your doctor should monitor your liver function carefully.

Niacin makes your liver work harder, so some elevated liver function is to be expected and isn't always the sign of a problem. I've heard about some doctors (not lipid specialists) pulling their patients off niacin because of concern about this issue. While this needs to be judged on a patient-to-patient basis, I will generally accept up to two times normal liver function in my patients on niacin if they have no symptoms.

Eyesight Change

In rare cases, niacin causes a change in the back part of the eye. You may perceive this as a change in your visual acuity. If this occurs, inform your doctor and a simple eye exam can determine if this is the problem or not. Most of the time this problem resolves when the niacin is discontinued.

Skin Conditions

Niacin can cause a temporary skin rash that is due to the enlargement of the blood vessels in the skin. This results in redness and can cause itching as well. This flushing is very common, and we'll discuss ways to fight back. Another skin condition is called acanthosis nigricans and can cause an increase in the pigmentation in the skin, most often in the armpits and groin.

Help with Minor Side Effects

The most common complaint we hear when treating patients with niacin is skin flushing. The drug can cause a tingling redness and discomfort in the face, neck, chest, and back. It's certainly uncomfortable, but it generally lasts 10 to 20 minutes and has no serious health consequences. This side effect often gets better the longer you are on niacin.

This is definitely a drug that patients need some assistance in managing, but it's so wonderfully effective, so inexpensive, and so relatively safe that I really do think it's worth the extra work.

One day I asked Dr. David Blankenhorn of the University of Southern California, one of the giants in this field, how he got his patients who had already undergone coronary artery bypass surgery to tolerate such high doses of niacin. He said, "I get them to open their shirts and ask them if they want another scar to match the one they've got." When the discomfort associated with flushing is put in perspective, it's much easier to convince someone to try some of the tricks we've learned to make it tolerable.

Because niacin *can* be managed. I helped design a fascinating study at Kaiser Permanente Medical Center in the San Francisco area. Patients with coronary heart disease were separated into two groups: One was sent back to their doctors and got normal care for their blood lipids, and the other group checked in monthly at a clinic staffed by nurses that I had trained to treat the patients using specific clinical pathways with little or no help from physicians. The nurses did much, much better than the doctors at improving the patients' blood lipids.

Why? Because their patients were more compliant with the treatments. They had a support system in the specially trained nurses, who had more time, patience, and tools than the doctors in the study. Let's say two patients on niacin experienced flushing. One would call his doctor, and the doctor would say, "Okay, it's not working out, forget about it, we'll try something else."

But the other patient would call the nurse, and she'd jolly him through it: "I'm sorry you're uncomfortable. Did you take an aspirin with it? Because sometimes that helps. What did you have for lunch? Chinese food? Well, there's your problem. All that hot, spicy stuff dilates your blood vessels so you're more likely to flush. Stay away from the Szechuan and call me back if you flush after your next dose, and maybe we'll drop you down to a lower dose for a little while." Of course, the patients who had access to the nurses, with all their little tricks and encouragements, had a greater likelihood of staying on the drug—and of improving their health. By the end of a year, about 20 percent of the doctors' patients were still on the drug—compared to about 90 percent of the nurses'.

Over the years, we've learned a lot of ways to make niacin therapy more comfortable, and I'd like to share some of them. Think of this section as your very own lipid nurse on call! This therapy is so good—so effective, so inexpensive, and so relatively safe—that it deserves the best chance we can give it. Remember: This must be done only under a physician's supervision.

Titrate

In order to minimize the side effects of niacin, we titrate, or build the dose slowly, starting at a very low dose and gradually increasing it until we get you to the target dose. This allows your body to get used to the drug and can help to minimize its reaction to it. We also recommend that our patients taking immediate-release niacin split the dose into two or three treatments over the course of the day, so that they're not taking the full dose at one fell swoop.

Take It with Food

Taking your niacin (and most drugs) with food helps to blunt the gastrointestinal side effects and may help to minimize the other side effects you experience. But any food that can make you flush exacerbates the flushing effect of niacin. This includes Chinese and Mexican foods, spicy foods, alcohol, and coffee.

Take a Baby Aspirin

Prostaglandin, the chemical that causes flushing, hangs out on the blood platelets. Aspirin slightly poisons platelets. So if you take a baby aspirin 20 or 30 minutes before you take your niacin, you should notice a reduction in flushing. You'll probably only need to take the aspirin as you're gradually increasing the dosage of niacin. When you arrive at the dose you're going to stay at, you can stop the aspirin after several days—your body will gradually adapt to the niacin dose, and your platelet response will change of its own accord.

Take It with Psyllium

One of our patients was having a hard time with flushing and gastrointestinal distress. He was also taking Metamucil for constipation, and he noticed that when he took the two together, he experienced a significant reduction in his symptoms from the niacin. The Metamucil probably decreases the rate of absorption of the niacin. Increasing your fiber intake is a good idea anyway.

Avoid Vasodilators

Avoid anything that will cause your blood vessels to dilate. Spicy foods are particularly bad, and Chinese food packs a double whammy: It's not only spicy, but it's often loaded with MSG, which is a powerful vasodilator on its own. Alcohol and caffeine can also cause problems—many of our patients notice reactions after their morning coffee or a glass of wine with dinner. Hot beverages (and hot baths) are also vasodilators, so avoid them when you take your niacin.

These tricks should help, and your physician (or nurse) may have other helpful tips. For the most part, the side effects of this drug are manageable. If you're doing everything right and you're still having difficulty with side effects, consider talking to your doctor about a slightly reduced dose.

Contraindications

As with every drug, there are people who are better not to take niacin. Here are some of the contraindications.

For Diabetics

Niacin may raise blood sugar and your insulin level. This occurs mostly in people who have high blood sugar and high insulin levels to begin with. In people who don't already have trouble with their blood sugar, we don't worry about this too much. In people who do, we tend to weigh the consequences: In your case, will the benefits of the niacin outweigh the problems associated with high levels of insulin? Niacin dosages are considerably lower than they used to be, and we see the blood sugar problem much less often now. And a number of very convincing recent studies have shown that diabetics can tolerate niacin very well with proper management.

As you probably know, most people with diabetes end up dying of coronary heart disease. Atherosclerosis is such an atrocious problem in people with diabetes (and prediabetic conditions) that my impulse is always to control the coronary heart disease as much as we possibly can and treat the insulin resistance with exercise and diet (and low-dose drugs, if necessary). As usual, the best policy is to monitor everything closely for a little while and to offer individualized treatment. If your insulin levels go up, but you're losing weight, then the benefits might outweigh the negatives. If your insulin goes up, and you don't or can't get your lifestyle issues under control, then you may want to cut the dose of niacin or try a fibrate, which won't raise your insulin. Niacin can also be combined with some of the more modern diabetes drugs to avoid the blood sugar and insulin issue.

For People with High Homocysteine

A study I conducted showed that niacin can raise homocysteine levels in some but not all people. This tends to be dose dependent—the higher the dose, the higher the homocysteine. In 60 percent of the people in the study, niacin had no effect on their homocysteine levels. In 40 percent of them, it did raise their homocysteine levels. The average was about two units—what that tells us is that in some people it hardly budged, and in some it went up a lot more. If you're one of the people whose homocysteine gets much higher when you're put on niacin, then it will show up in your blood work, and your doctor can make a correction accordingly. In most cases, he or she will add a B vitamin to lower the homocysteine. Correcting the lipid disorder trumps regulating the homocysteine naturally.

For People with Peptic Ulcers

Niacin should not be taken by people who have an active peptic ulcer.

Other Benefits

Niacin decreases vasoreactivity. It decreases fibrinogen levels, and while it's not an anticoagulant, it discourages certain kinds of clotting and platelet stickiness. It may also lower hs-CRP and is one of the few drugs that appear to have an effect on Lp(a).

FIBRATES

The other set of drugs in this plan is the fibrates. Although we have lots of strategies for dealing with niacin's tricky side effects, some people truly can't tolerate them. They may also have underlying medical conditions, like gout or an ulcer, that make niacin an untenable choice. If that's the case, then we usually try fibrates.

Common Names

These drugs are also called fibric acid derivatives. Some brand names include clofibrate (Atromid-S), fenofibrate (Tricor), and gemfibrozil (Lopid).

What They Do

The fibrates are especially good at lowering triglycerides (by 30 to 50 percent). They may or may not lower LDL. Gemfibrozil may increase LDL-C slightly, and fenofibrate lowers LDL-C slightly. Fibrates tend to raise HDL-C, particularly when a problem with elevated triglycerides is reduced by the fibrate. They may also lower hs-CRP and fibrinogen.

The fibrates work especially well on people who have high triglycerides and low HDL—in fact, it is a perfect match for these individuals.

How They Work

If you're taking a fibrate, you're actually doing gene manipulation.

The way the fibrates work is by going to your genetic material and essentially flipping a switch. They tell the gene that produces that magic enzyme LPL to make more of it. This enzyme chews up triglycerides, and that's why the fibrates are so good at lowering triglycerides. The fibrates also go to the gene that produces one of the essential building blocks for HDL, and they tell it to make more blocks, which is how they raise HDL. In other words, they go to the genes and tell them to turn up the heat on things that benefit coronary heart disease (such as HDL production) and to turn down the heat on things that contribute to coronary heart disease, like high triglycerides.

The end result is a supercharged metabolic system that gets rid of triglycerides and increases HDL production.

Side Effects

Here are some side effects to watch out for if you're taking a fibrate.

Gastrointestinal Distress

You may experience some gastrointestinal distress while you're taking the fibrates, including gas, constipation, and upset stomach. Drinking lots of water and increasing the fiber in your diet helps.

Gallstones

Some of the older fibrates, such as clofibrate, have been associated with an increased risk of gallstone formation, but this has not been reported with the newer fibrate, fenofibrate.

Muscle Inflammation

Muscle inflammation, or myositis, may occur with these medications just like we described in the statin section.

To recap, this is a relatively rare and potentially serious side effect, which feels like muscle pain or discomfort—the kind you feel after a vigorous workout—or when you're coming down with the flu. It's uncomfortable and can be very serious, even resulting in kidney failure or death. If you think you have symptoms of myositis while on a fibrate, call your physician.

This has most commonly been reported with the older gemfibrozil and less with fenofibrate.

Bowel Cancer

Some of the older fibrates, such as clofibrate, were linked to an increased risk of bowel cancer, which is one of the reasons that they fell out of favor. This does not appear to be true of the newer fibrate drugs.

Contraindications

Although generally safe, it's not always appropriate to use the fibrates in the presence of other medications.

Combined with Statin Drugs

Some people have experienced kidney and muscle inflammation when combining fibrates with the statins. Your doctor may wish to test your blood periodically if you're on this combination to ensure that you're not having this problem.

May Enhance Effects of Blood Thinners

Many heart patients are on blood thinners derived from Coumadin or warfarin. The fibrates can make these blood thinners work even better than they are supposed to and the end result may be blood that is too thin, and dangerously so. If you are on one of these blood thinners and then placed on a fibrate, your physician will likely reduce the dose of the blood thinner.

Other Benefits

The fibrates also improve vasoreactivity and have been reported to lower hs-CRP. They also lower fibrinogen, so they may prevent a tendency toward abnormal blood clotting in people with high fibrinogen levels.

THE NIACIN-FIBRATE COMBINATION

Since niacin and fibrates work to increase HDL in two totally different ways, we can get some brilliant results by combining them.

Fibrates tell the gene to make more building blocks, and niacin keeps the resulting HDL from degrading, which means that you're receiving its beneficial effects a lot longer. So these two drugs used in combination with one another can really raise your HDL, your "good" cholesterol.

MEDICATION PLAN #2:
THE HEAVYWEIGHT PLAN

Niacin, Fibrate, or Niacin + Fibrate
It is only appropriate to take medication under the supervision of a physician.

OTHER MEDICATIONS THAT MAY HELP YOUR HEART: DIABETES MEDICATION

Some commonly prescribed diabetes medications have been shown to increase beneficial HDL cholesterol, lower triglycerides, and to help with the LDL subclass issue as well. One of these drugs is metformin; other beneficial medications include the group of drugs called the thiazolidine-diones. The sulfonylureas, which are the other commonly prescribed group, don't have the same beneficial effects. If you've been diagnosed with elevated blood sugar, you'll want to have a conversation with your doctor about the relative benefits of these medications.

MEDICATION PLAN #3
THE ONE-TWO PUNCH PLAN

This plan is designed for people with elevated apo B and at least one *other* metabolic disorder. It uses the statin drugs plus another drug, either niacin or a fibrate. The statin drug treats the apo B, and the second drug will address the other metabolic disorder, depending on which one it is.

Where multiple low-dose therapies are possible, I like to use them. You get the same result, but you're on lower doses of each drug and therefore are less likely to experience side effects from either of them.

Who Should Follow This Medication Plan?

- People with elevated apo B *and* at least one of the other three metabolic disorders in the Medication Prescription Key

Statin-Niacin Combinations

As far as combination therapies go, this statin-niacin combination is breathtakingly effective. The drug companies are starting to get savvy to it and have actually started to market a combination drug that enables the patient to do

Timing Tip

When you're using statins in combination with fibrates, separate the doses. Take your fibrate in the morning and your statin in the evening, and you'll be less likely to experience an interaction between the two.

a little end run around the insurance companies (you only have to pay one prescription copay instead of two).

Niacin-resin combinations are also very successful. In fact, the first study to show that coronary heart disease is reversible, the University of Southern California's Cholesterol Lowering Atherosclerosis Study, studied men after coronary artery bypass surgery and used a niacin-resin combination.

Statin-Fibrate Combinations

The results of this combination are very similar to the results you see when a statin drug is used in combination with niacin. The principal difference is that the statin-niacin combination has been used in a great number of clinical trials. On the other hand, the fibrates tend to be a little better tolerated than niacin, so if someone has medical conditions (like elevated uric acid) that contraindicate the niacin, or if they've had a really hard time with the side effects of the niacin, then a statin-fibrate combination is something to consider.

The only thing to watch out for here is that the statin-fibrate combination raises your risk of myositis, that muscle inflammation that can have such serious consequences. Again, this really highlights why medication therapy has to be done under close medical supervision.

MEDICATION PLAN #3:
THE ONE-TWO PUNCH PLAN

Statin + Niacin or Statin + Fibrate
It is only appropriate to take medication under the supervision of a physician.

A NOTE ABOUT BETA-BLOCKERS

You're probably familiar with beta-blockers, which are a popular and very effective way to treat hypertension. Beta-blockers can have some unpleasant effects on your lipid profile. These drugs may elevate triglycerides, lower beneficial HDL cholesterol, and exacerbate the LDL pattern B issue.

There's another class of drugs, called alpha-blockers, which can also be used to treat hypertension, and they have the opposite effect: They lower triglycerides, raise beneficial HDL, and can help to convert people from LDL pattern B to LDL pattern A. All good stuff! If you have this small LDL pattern B issue and you're taking a beta-blocker to control your blood pressure, you may want to discuss the possibility of switching to an alpha-blocker with your physician.

You can see now why I consider these Advanced Metabolic Markers such an enormous leap forward in the way we treat cardiac disease. These blood tests not only aid in prevention, but they enable us to use the medications we already have in a targeted, precise way to treat a multitude of underlying metabolic problems. The results in both instances are far reaching and have afforded doctors and their patients an unprecedented opportunity to reverse this disease.

10

THE SUPPLEMENT
PRESCRIPTION

AN INTRODUCTION TO SUPPLEMENTS AND YOUR HEART

TAKING SUPPLEMENTS TO IMPROVE your heart health has received a considerable amount of public attention in the last two decades. While there isn't an abundance of sound scientific data with which to judge the usefulness and safety of supplements, I do believe that in certain circumstances they can be a valuable Prescription as part of a full-spectrum heart health program.

WHAT'S A SUPPLEMENT?

A supplement is anything taken to augment, or supplement, the diet. The body doesn't make its own vitamins and minerals—it takes what it needs from the foods we eat. If the foods that we eat don't supply enough of those vitamins and minerals or if some aspect of our lives overtaxes our supply of those things, supplements can be taken to make up for the deficiency.

Vitamins often act as turbochargers for the chemical reactions that go on in the body. It's also important to note that, unlike essential amino acids or fatty acids, only very small amounts of vitamins are necessary to sustain life. The real question is how much of these supplements are optimal for cardiovascular health.

Whether alone or in combination with some of the medications we discussed in the last chapter, many of these supplements may contribute to the prevention and treatment of coronary heart disease. In this chapter, we'll go through the most effective ones: what they are, what they do, how they do it, what research supports them, the side effects or possible drug reactions that have been reported, as well as my own recommendations for their use.

And since there are so many supplements out there being touted as miracle cures for coronary heart disease, I thought I'd weigh in on some of the most popular. If you walk into a supplement store and tell them you're worried about coronary heart disease, they'll happily fill a basket full of supplements for you—but what's really in there? My patients are always bringing me articles and asking me questions about specific over-the-counter remedies, and I thought it would be helpful to review some of the supplements most commonly reported to help with atherosclerosis and coronary heart disease. I've broken these down into three categories: Possibly Helpful, Unclear, and Possibly Harmful.

Treat Supplements like Medicine

I'd like to begin our discussion of supplements with a warning. There's a common misconception that vitamins, minerals, and herbs are harmless simply because they're "natural" products. This simply isn't true. While these supplements can be very effective in affecting your cardiac profile, they can also be toxic in the incorrect dosage, they can react badly with other medications you're taking, and they can have harmful effects on other aspects of your health.

It's important to remember that we don't have either the safety or the efficacy data on supplements like we do on the FDA-approved drugs. Nobody has conducted the kind of large, placebo-controlled studies we'd need to determine their effectiveness or side effects because these studies are very, very expensive to conduct. So there are always question marks when we're dealing with supplements—there's simply not a lot of hard information out there about them.

Just because supplements are available without a doctor's prescription at the drugstore doesn't mean that you should take them without medical supervision; please do not begin taking supplements until you've discussed the specific supplement *and dosage* with your doctor.

You may also want to get your doctor's specific recommendation about brand names. All supplements are not created equal: Since they're not regulated by the FDA, there can be a truly shocking lack of consistency in their makeup and potency.

The Best Supplement of All: A Healthy, Well-Balanced Diet

Your mother was right: Much of what we need to stay healthy can be obtained from a well-balanced diet.

Many of the supplements we'll discuss in this chapter are available naturally from food sources. And many of the beneficial foods that we discussed in the nutrition chapter—things like soy and the importance of fiber—might also count as supplements. This serves to remind us once more that what you put into your mouth directly affects your health. A well-varied diet that's rich in fruits and vegetables will go a long way toward keeping you healthy.

AN ASPIRIN A DAY MAY KEEP THE CARDIOLOGIST AWAY

I recommend to my patients that they take a baby aspirin every day if there are no medical contraindications. If you're at risk for coronary heart disease, you should talk to your doctor to find out if he thinks it's a good idea for you.

Aspirin works to decrease your blood's tendency to clot. Platelets are components in your blood that aid with clotting and the "stickiness" of your blood. That's ordinarily a good thing; it prevents you from bleeding to death from a paper cut, for instance. But as we know, thrombosis, or blood clots that get stuck around the plaque in the arteries, are a major cause of heart attack. So it benefits people with coronary heart disease to decrease platelet aggregation, or stickiness. Aspirin reduces the blood's clotting tendency by poisoning some of those platelets.

At a recent American Heart Association scientific meeting, investigators reported that aspirin can also lower Lp(a) a little bit.

Since it's an inexpensive treatment with few serious side effects, I do recommend that people at risk for coronary heart disease take a baby aspirin a day. Consult with your doctor to ensure that he agrees. **There are people who shouldn't take aspirin, and you'll want to make certain that you're not one of them.**

Aspirin and High-Sensitivity C-Reactive Protein

My general aspirin recommendation is more than a general recommendation for my patients with elevated high-sensitivity C-reactive protein (hs-CRP). As anyone who's ever used aspirin for a headache or muscle pain after a hard workout knows, aspirin also acts as an anti-inflammatory. As you'll remember, hs-CRP is an indicator that there's inflammation in your system. Since inflammation contributes to coronary heart disease by weakening and destabilizing the fatty buildup inside the arterial walls, causing rupture and blood clots, taking anti-inflammatory measures may be a good way to prevent heart attack and stroke.

In one large study of physicians conducted through Harvard University, the physicians who took aspirin were shown to have significantly fewer heart attacks compared to the physicians who did not take aspirin. However, in later analysis, it was discovered that the greatest benefit of aspirin was in preventing heart attacks in the physicians who also had elevated hs-CRP. So if my patients have elevated hs-CRP and there's no reason why they shouldn't be taking aspirin, I recommend it.

Aspirin: Contraindications

Everyone should check in with their doctor before beginning any kind of therapy, and a daily baby aspirin—no matter how harmless it might seem—is no exception. People with gastrointestinal problems such as stomach bleeding or ulcers and anyone with an allergy to aspirin should never go on aspirin therapy.

THE SUPPLEMENT PLANS

As with the Nutrition, Exercise, and Medication components of this program, you'll use the Prescription Key on page 289 to help you locate the individualized Supplement Plan that has been calibrated to meet the needs of your particular cardiac profile. All you'll need to do is match the results of your own tests against the Prescription Key to find the plan that is right for you.

Our first plan is the **Antioxidant Defense Plan**. If your blood work indicates that you're at risk from oxidative damage, then simple vitamin therapy can provide you with essential fortification at the cellular level. The next plan is the **Fish Oil Rx Plan**. The essential fatty acids in cold-water fish like salmon have an astonishingly positive effect on heart health, but it's hard to get what you need from a sardine sandwich. This plan explores those benefits and the benefits conferred by a more concentrated supplemental dose. The third and final plan is the **Homocysteine Solution Plan**. Again, here we'll use simple vitamin therapy to rally your body's natural defenses—in this case, to bolster the enzyme that ordinarily helps boost your body's own ability to cleanse itself of this atherogenic chemical.

So which of these plans do you need?

Using the Prescription Key

Directly below the Supplement Prescription Key on page 289 you'll see a list of four markers labeled "My Supplement Markers." These will determine which individualized Supplement Plan is the right fit for your cardiac profile.

Refer back to your Quick Reference Chart on page 91 to help you to fill in a "yes" or "no" in the space provided beside each Supplement Marker. (Let's do an example together: Harriet has tested "normal" on Lp(a), LDL pattern B, and homocysteine, and "abnormal" on triglycerides, so her column would read "No," "No," "No," "Yes.")

Once you have your list of yeses and no's, just look up at the Key and find the column that duplicates your pattern. (Remember, read down the columns, from top to bottom, until you find your exact match.)

At the base of the column that matches your own results, you'll find the number that identifies *your* plan. (Harriet would find the plan that matches her pattern in the 11th column from the left. Since the number at the base of the column is 2, she should proceed to the second Supplement Plan, the Fish Oil Rx Plan.)

So refer back to your Quick Reference chart on page 91, and let's get started!

Note #1: You'll notice that this Supplement Prescription Key works a little differently than the other Keys in this book. In some cases within this Key, you'll be guided to *more than one* Supplement Plan. That's because your combination of metabolic markers indicates that you could benefit from following more than one Supplement Plan. Don't worry: These plans all complement each other and can be used in combination with one another, so there's no fear of conflict.

Note #2: Please do not begin taking supplements until you've discussed the specific supplement *and dosage* with your doctor.

Note #3: If you haven't taken the Advanced Metabolic Marker tests, or if you're still waiting for your results, don't worry. Even though we can't direct you to a Supplement Plan, you can still gain plenty of information by reading through the plans. In my practice I won't prescribe medications or supplements for my patients before carefully analyzing their Advanced Metabolic Marker tests. I can't in good faith treat my patients without this additional knowledge, and I can't make recommendations to you here about supplements unless you know the status of your own advanced markers.

That said, even without the testing, there's plenty for you to do in order to begin your journey down the road to lifelong heart health. Be sure to follow the Nutrition and Exercise Prescriptions that have been assigned to you! If you decide to get tested in the future, then you'll be able to insert your numbers into the Prescription Key and find out which Supplement Plan is right for you.

The Supplement Prescription Key

Supplement Marker														
Lp(a)	Yes	Yes	Yes	Yes	Yes	Yes	No	No	No	No	No	No	No	No
LDL pattern B	No	Yes	No	No	No	Yes	Yes	No	No	No	Yes	Yes	Yes	No
Homocysteine	No	Yes	Yes	No	Yes	Yes	Yes	Yes	No	No	No	Yes	No	Yes
Triglycerides	No	No	No	Yes	Yes	Yes	Yes	Yes	Yes	No	Yes	No	No	No
Supplement Plan #:	1	1,3	1,3	1,2	1,2,3	1,2,3	1,2,3	2,3	2	N/A	1,2	1,3	1	3

Supplement Plan #1: THE ANTIOXIDANT DEFENSE PLAN

Supplement Plan #2: THE FISH OIL RX PLAN

Supplement Plan #3: THE HOMOCYSTEINE SOLUTION PLAN

My Supplement Markers:

Lp(a) _____

LDL pattern B _____

Homocysteine _____

Triglycerides _____

SUPPLEMENT PLAN #1
THE ANTIOXIDANT DEFENSE PLAN

In this plan, nature's housekeepers come to the rescue. The two supplements we use in this plan, vitamin C and vitamin E, can prevent oxidation, one of the first steps in the formation of atherosclerosis and unstable plaque.

What is oxidation?

To understand why antioxidants are so important, we need a refresher course in the dangers of oxidation.

Rust is a form of oxidation. So is the browning of the flesh of an apple when it's cut and exposed to the air. These two examples demonstrate that although oxygen is a necessity, it has potentially damaging effects as well. For instance, it can have a very damaging "rusting" effect on certain proteins attached to the LDL particles, like apo B and Lp(a). This damage changes the shape of these proteins, and as you'll see, that change is *extremely* dangerous. To understand why, we have to understand a little about the relationship between "oxidized" LDL and the white blood cells that protect the arteries.

Oxidized LDL and Plaque Instability

Macrophages, or the white blood cells, are the body's natural defense system, and they're everywhere, including in the walls of the arteries. They work like vacuum cleaners, using their aptly named scavenger receptors to detect potentially dangerous interlopers in the walls of your arteries. When they find something that shouldn't be there, the receptors sound an alarm and the white blood cell scavenges, or gobbles up, the offending intruder.

Now, most cells with other types of receptors have a turn-off switch. It's an internal safety measure to prevent the cell from gorging itself to death, like feeling sick when we eat too much—that's the signal to stop eating before the stomach explodes. In the same way, when these cells hit a certain threshold, the receptors turn themselves off.

There's only one problem. Unlike other types of cells with receptor mechanisms, these macrophages don't have a turn-off switch. They *can't* turn themselves off. So the white blood cell never gets the message to stop eating. It eats and eats until it becomes obese, turning into what's called a foam cell, because the fats inside have the appearance of foam. Foam cells are unstable and prone to pop. When they do, that can rupture the arterial plaque. This is a gross over-simplification of the process, but if you imagine a water balloon filled to bursting, you've got the general idea of what happens to the foam cells in the arterial walls. And they're lethal—when the plaque ruptures, it can completely obstruct a partially blocked artery, causing a heart attack and even sudden death.

So what's the connection to oxidization? The key is in the change that happens in the particles attached to the LDL. When these particles are oxidized, the LDL becomes *especially* attractive to the white blood cell's scavenger receptor. These unregulated macrophages gobble oxidized LDL up like candy. So the chemical process of oxidation accelerates the whole process: The macrophages eat more and more of these oxidized LDL, become obese foam cells, the foam cells get even fatter, and they explode—and all of this is happening much faster than it would if we were dealing with ordinary LDL. In this way, oxidation increases the likelihood of arterial damage, unstable plaque, and a cardiac event.

Obviously, we're looking to do anything we can to shore up the body's natural defenses against this perilous process. And the antioxidants in this plan are one way to do that. Now, antioxidants won't change your blood-work numbers like some of the other supplements will, but there's quite a bit of evidence to suggest that they can have a protective effect in many people. Because there isn't a drug company behind these supplements, it's hard to get

Who Should Use This Supplement Plan?

- People with LDL pattern B
- People with high triglycerides
- People with high Lp(a)
- People with low HDL2b
- People who smoke

the funding to obtain good clinical data to determine how effective they truly are. But since they're inexpensive and have a very low incidence of side effects (none of my patients have ever had an adverse reaction), I do suggest these antioxidant supplements for people whose blood tests suggest that they're susceptible to oxidative damage.

People with LDL Pattern B

People with small LDLs are at especially high risk for oxidation for a very simple reason: Research conducted at the University of California by Dr. Tribble and Dr. Krauss has shown that they have lipoprotein particles that are much more susceptible to oxidative damage because they carry fewer natural antioxidants.

People with High Triglycerides

It's for this same reason that people with high triglycerides are in danger from oxidation. Triglycerides are carried around in very-low-density lipoproteins (VLDLs), particles that are inherently susceptible to oxidation. And people who have high triglycerides have a lot of these VLDLs and intermediate-density lipoproteins, which means that they're at *extra* risk—not only do they have these particles in their bloodstreams, but they have a lot of them.

People with High Lp(a)

People with elevated levels of Lp(a) are at high risk for oxidative damage. Again, the reason why is part of the oxidized LDL story: Lp(a) is one of the proteins that can be attached to the LDL particle in some people. When this protein becomes oxidized, it changes shape, and that new shape is very attractive to that scavenger receptor on the white blood cells.

In 1989, Dr. Margaret Haberland and colleagues conducted experiments that showed that oxidized Lp(a) caused the foam cells to eat LDL 60 times faster than normal, a positively staggering increase. So people with a lot of Lp(a) may be at higher risk than others from the dangers of oxidation.

People with Low HDL2b

Unlike LDL, HDL comes with its own antioxidant shield. In fact, one of the best antioxidants out there is one you can't buy: It's produced by the body.

It's called paraoxanase, and it lives on HDL2b, so when HDL2b is high, paraoxanase is high, and it provides a very high degree of natural antioxidant protection. Conversely, when HDL2b is low, paraoxanase is low, which means that you're at high risk for oxidative damage. So raising your HDL2b not only helps with reverse cholesterol transport, the beneficial process by which cholesterol is removed from arterial plaque and returned to the liver for recycling, but it automatically increases your body's natural defense against oxidization. If your HDL2b is low, then adding antioxidant supplements may bolster your body's ability to resist oxidation.

As I'll discuss in greater detail later, a recent study showed that antioxidants blunt the HDL-raising effects of niacin. So if you're on niacin to raise your HDL, you and your doctor may decide not to use antioxidants.

People Who Smoke

The worst oxidant out there is ozone, so people whose work involves exhaust or air pollution, like highway patrol officers, factory workers who come in constant contact with fumes, and car mechanics may be at higher risk due to exposure to ozone air pollution. Several years ago I conducted experiments at the University of California, Davis, in which patients with coronary artery disease ran on a treadmill while breathing air with different concentrations of ozone in it. High concentrations of ozone brought angina on sooner than the lower doses.

The second worst oxidant is cigarette smoke, which is literally filled with tons of oxidative by-products. Every cigarette you smoke oxidizes your cells like crazy, and if you're a pack-a-day smoker, you're doing it 20 times a day. Smokers, therefore, are at extremely high risk of oxidative damage and might benefit from antioxidant supplementation.

Note: Vitamin E may have other adverse affects in smokers, so you should absolutely check with your doctor before beginning an antioxidant program.

So now we know who's likely to benefit from antioxidants. We've enlisted two supplements for their antioxidant effects: vitamins C and E. Let's take a closer look at their properties.

VITAMIN E (ALPHATOCOPHEROL)

Alphatocopherol and other antioxidants are actually carried within the LDL and other lipoprotein particles. The more tocopherol (vitamin E) there is within the LDL particle, the more resistant it is to oxidative damage. That's a good thing, since oxidized LDL can be so lethal.

Does vitamin E work?

What evidence is there that vitamin E works? There is currently a very interesting debate regarding the potential benefit of antioxidant supplements. The basic science is quite clear but, unfortunately, the clinical science remains cloudy. The Cambridge Heart Attack and Antioxidant Study (CHAOS) showed that men with coronary heart disease who took vitamin E showed a significant reduction in nonfatal heart attacks. This study strongly suggested that vitamin E is beneficial if you already have coronary heart disease.

But, like all supplement therapy, vitamin E is not without controversy. As with drug therapy, you want two or three studies that show similar results. In a drug trial, researchers gave the control group doses of vitamin E and saw no reduction in cardiovascular events, which led them to conclude that E doesn't work to reduce heart attack risk. Of course, they weren't looking specifically at people who are at risk for oxidative damage; rather than giving vitamin E to all comers, it makes sense to think that it would be most beneficial in patients with a susceptibility to that particular damage.

More suspicion was thrown on the issue when Dr. Greg Brown at the University of Washington in Seattle completed a research study that included the use of antioxidants (vitamins C and E, beta-carotene, and selenium) with the lipid drugs niacin and simvastatin. The niacin and simvastatin without antioxidants significantly improved coronary artery measurements of how much obstruction the patients had and resulted in an astonishing 89 percent reduction in clinical events. Unfortunately, the group that got the antioxidant mix as well as the medications had significantly less benefit in regard to obstruction improvement and had more clinical events. And the antioxidant supplements appeared to blunt the beneficial effect that niacin had on increasing HDL-C and HDL2b.

How do I interpret the results of these studies? In the case of Dr. Brown's study, if I am attempting to raise HDL-C with niacin in a patient already taking vitamins E and C, and the HDL-C does not go up as expected, the first option is to increase the dose of niacin. The second option is to stop the vitamins C and E and see if that increases HDL-C without increasing the dose of niacin.

Most recently, a study was completed at the University of Southern California called Vitamin E Atherosclerosis Prevention Study (VEAPS). This was a well-designed study that investigated the effect of vitamin E on the thickness of the carotid artery wall. The hope was to prevent progression of atherosclerosis in the carotid artery, but the initial report indicates that there was no benefit from the vitamin E treatment.

So the scientific justification to take vitamin E in order to protect the heart has taken several blows recently. We have always used the antioxidant vitamins only in patients susceptible to oxidative damage, which includes those with elevated Lp(a) and an abundance of small LDL, or a deficiency of HDL. The decision to use antioxidant vitamins is now a tricky one. If you and your physician decide that you should take antioxidant vitamins, I suggest that you keep a close eye on your HDL-C and HDL2b levels. If they don't go up as expected, or perhaps even go down, you and your physician will want to consider stopping the antioxidants. Hopefully, future research will identify the types of people who are likely to benefit from these vitamins.

VITAMIN C (ASCORBIC ACID)

You may remember the example of the cut apple flesh that turns brown unless sprinkled with lemon juice. In that case, it's the vitamin C in the lemon juice that protects the apple flesh from oxidization.

Vitamin C is, in fact, one of our most powerful antioxidants. Dr. Linus Pauling is best known for his elucidation of the nature of the chemical bond, work for which he won the Nobel Prize. His work on vitamin C is really wonderful science, even though it has been misunderstood in many instances by the popular media. Dr. Pauling noted that every animal in the world produces vitamin C naturally, except for the primates: monkeys, humans, and the guinea pig. He figured out approximately how much vitamin C other animals were making, and based on body mass, extrapolated that humans should be getting

Supplement to Avoid: Beta-Carotene

For years, the antioxidant supplements we used to defend against coronary heart disease were vitamin C, vitamin E, and beta-carotene, a precursor to vitamin A. As you can see, we're still considering the use of vitamin C and E, but beta-carotene has fallen off the list. The reason: In a major study, beta-carotene appeared to be linked to an increase in cancer among smokers. So while we no longer suggest that our patients take beta-carotene supplements, we still recommend that people eat foods rich in this vitamin, like sweet potatoes, carrots, cantaloupe, squash, apricot, and mango—all yellow-orange in color, you'll notice. The dark leafy greens, including vegetables like spinach, collard greens, and kale, are also good sources of beta-carotene.

much more vitamin C a day than we normally do. Now, if you're a monkey and all you do is eat jungle fruit all day, you're probably getting something close to that. If you're a human and your vitamin C intake is limited to grabbing a glass of O.J. in the morning (if you're lucky), you're not getting anywhere close to the amount you should be getting.

One of the functions of vitamin C is to enable the construction of a certain kind of amino acid called **hydroxyproline**. Dr. Pauling believed that in order for the body to fight insults to it such as infection, additional vitamin C would be helpful by increasing the body's ability to produce this important amino acid.

A Winning Combination

Vitamin C and vitamin E are particularly powerful when working together. Vitamin E gets changed in the antioxidation process, which decreases its usefulness, but vitamin C can help to rejuvenate that used-up vitamin E, reinvigorating it with antioxidant properties, so you'll get more bang for your vitamin E buck when you combine the two.

SUPPLEMENT PLAN #1: THE ANTIOXIDANT DEFENSE PLAN

Take 400 IU of vitamin E and 500 milligrams of vitamin C every day.

SUPPLEMENT PLAN #2
THE FISH OIL RX PLAN

Your choice of entrée may have a greater impact on your heart health than you know! We're discovering that the fatty acids in fish have a profound effect on your cardiac health, and the more concentrated doses available in fish oil supplements may be very beneficial for certain metabolic imbalances.

Who Should Use This Supplement Plan?

- People with high triglycerides
- People with high blood pressure
- People with LDL pattern B
- People with existing coronary heart disease

People with High Triglycerides

The traditional use of fish oils for many years has been to lower very high triglycerides.

In patients with triglycerides in the 1,000 range, these can have a significantly beneficial effect—and these patients also sometimes show an increase in HDL-C. In patients with moderately high triglycerides, fish oil supplements have been shown to reduce the triglycerides, but in these patients, HDL-C was also reduced, which is not what we like to see.

In general, the higher your triglycerides are, the better the effects.

People with High Blood Pressure

Fish oils have also been used to help treat high blood pressure. In patients with mild hypertension, 6 grams a day of fish oil reduced the systolic blood pressure by about 5 millimeters of mercury (mm Hg) and the diastolic by 3 mm Hg. Interestingly enough, in this study, the people who were already eating three or more fish meals a week had no blood pressure benefit from the supplementation.

People with LDL Pattern B

As you know, the fish oils are strongly associated with reduced triglycerides, and it's in that capacity that they're associated with a reduction in small LDL—it's a seesaw effect. As you remember, lipoprotein lipase's evil twin, hepatic lipase, controls the expression of the small LDL trait; the more hepatic lipase there is, the more small LDL there will be. The two enzymes work in opposition to one another: When lipoprotein lipase goes up, hepatic lipase goes down. So when there's a lot of lipoprotein lipase out there lowering triglycerides, there's less hepatic lipase to promote small LDL.

People with Existing Coronary Heart Disease

We're only beginning to understand how these oils work their magic on your heart, but what we do know leads me to believe that fish oils may be very beneficial for people with existing coronary heart disease.

Fish oils may help to prevent irregular heartbeats, possibly by helping to control the electrical impulses that control and stabilize heart rhythm. They help to maintain the elasticity of the artery walls, partially by inhibiting the synthesis of thromboxane, which is responsible for vasoconstriction. They integrate themselves into the arterial cell walls, helping to stabilize plaque that might otherwise have the potential to rupture. In some studies, they seem to help control angina, or chest pain, perhaps through some of the mechanisms we've already discussed.

They help to prevent platelet aggregation or "stickiness," which provides an anticoagulant effect a little bit like aspirin's. They inhibit the production of both apo B and very low-density lipoprotein and can help to convert LDL pattern B people to pattern As. There is also some slight evidence that these fats act as anti-inflammatory agents. Italian researchers discovered that survivors of heart attack significantly reduced both their chances of a second heart attack and of sudden death if they took omega-3s. These fatty acids may reduce the risk of heart attack if you suffer from angina, and they may reduce the severity of the heart attack if it comes.

THE FISH OIL STORY

Scientists first speculated about the benefits of fish oil after noticing that the Inuit Eskimos of Greenland had remarkably low incidence of coronary heart disease, despite a diet that was hugely high in fat. They also tended to bleed easily.

The fats the Inuits were eating came from whale, seal, and salmon, fish high in a class of polyunsaturated fatty acids called omega-3s, or n-3 polyunsaturated fatty acids, or the n-3 PUFAs. We discussed these in chapter 7. There are three kinds of omega-3s: eicosapentaenoic acid (EPA), docosahexaenoic acid (DHA), and alpha-linolenic acid (ALA). EPA and DHA are found in fish; ALA is found in some leafy greens and in flaxseed and does not have the same specific benefits. (Another class of these fatty acids, called omega-6s or n-6 PUFAs, does not have the same benefits as the omega-3s.)

The Inuits showed low levels of coronary heart disease and it was believed their fish oil–rich diet was protecting them.

Fish Oils Promote Heart Health

There's an overwhelming amount of scientific evidence, from studies done in animals and humans, that fish oils promote heart health. The Oslo Study Diet and Anti-Smoking Trial, which was done in 1,200 men by Dr. Hjermann in Norway, is one of the strongest arguments out there for super-effective therapy that doesn't involve drugs. The researchers saw a significant reduction in heart attack rate, and the only therapy they used was getting people to eat more fish and to stop smoking.

Another study was done in the Netherlands by Dr. Arntzenius and his colleagues, who looked at people with blocked coronary arteries and asked one group to eat between three and five fish meals a week, while the other group did nothing different. Five years later, there was a significant improvement in the arteries of the fish group—and again, no drugs were used.

And among the 85,000 women enrolled in the Nurses' Health Study conducted at Harvard University, those who ate fish two to four times per week reduced their risk of coronary heart disease by 30 percent, compared to women who rarely ate fish. The Physicians' Health Study, also conducted through Harvard University, showed that healthy men who got a lot of these omega-3 fatty acids by eating fish significantly reduced their chance of sudden coronary death.

And fish oils are also helpful for some kinds of irregular heartbeats and arterial spasms, although their exact role is still being investigated.

It's pretty compelling, isn't it? But there are some questions. Is the fish (oil) consumption itself what's making the difference? I have theorized that people who eat fish regularly are more health conscious in general—they tend to eat better and exercise more. The results may be overdetermined if the fish oils aren't the only contributing factor: In other words, was the benefit due to the fish they were eating or the fact that because they ate more fish, they ate less hamburger?

Things to Watch Out For

Mercury. Although fish has been an important food source for millennia and is unlikely to be toxic, there are some concerns. Unfortunately, today there are high levels of mercury and pesticides in fish due to the polluted waters they live in, and consumption of contaminated fish or fish oil can pass these poisons on to you. If you're taking a fish-oil supplement, make sure there's some indication on the label that the mercury levels have been checked in the oils used.

Excessive bleeding. Bleeding time can be prolonged with fish oils, and there is some concern about spontaneous bleeding, or excessive bleeding during surgery or after trauma. You should always consult with your physician before taking any kind of supplement, and if you're considering fish oils, you should specifically discuss this concern.

An omega-3 fat is still a fat. These fats are still fats, and that means that they're high in calories. If you're on a reduced-fat, reduced-calorie diet, you're going to have to examine the rest of your dietary intake and make accommodations for these supplements.

Cost of the supplement. These fish oil supplements are relatively expensive, and you have to take a lot of them, so that may be a consideration in your decision to pursue this supplementation path.

SUPPLEMENT PLAN #2:
THE FISH OIL RX PLAN

Take 3 to 6 grams of fish oils a day.

Fish is lower in saturated fat and calories than meat, so it's automatically a healthier protein choice. But the supposition that the fish oils are themselves beneficial comes with too much convincing science behind it for the "healthier diet" theory to be all there is to it. The American Heart Association recommends two servings of fish a week, at a minimum. Not all fish are created equal, though: Omega-3 levels are highest in fatty, cold-water fish, like mackerel, salmon, trout, tuna, sardines, and herring.

I believe that there are good basic science reasons to eat fish as often as possible and to supplement with concentrated doses of these oils if there's a metabolic reason to do so.

SUPPLEMENT PLAN #3
THE HOMOCYSTEINE SOLUTION PLAN

Homocysteine is a chemical produced in the body when the amino acid called methionine is metabolized. When levels in the blood are elevated, homocysteine signals a possible genetic predisposition toward coronary heart disease and is itself an arterial irritant. The best medicine to attack one of the most serious metabolic imbalances is a simple combination of vitamins.

Who Should Follow This Plan?

- People with high blood homocysteine

Homocysteine is a naturally occurring by-product of the amino acid methionine, which is made by the body in the process of digesting food, especially meat. Most people don't have a problem with this homocysteine: They eat some chicken, their homocysteine levels rise, and their bodies automatically flush the residual levels out of their bloodstreams.

But some people inherit either a compromised ability or a complete inability to clear homocysteine from their bloodstream, so their homocysteine levels remain high. Homocysteine itself is irritating to the inside of the arteries, acting almost like a piece of sandpaper. This not only causes inflammation but irritates the surface, making it easier for the other factors that cause coronary heart disease to worm their way into the arterial wall to do their damage.

So if you've inherited this inability to adequately clear homocysteine from your blood, your body needs additional support to get the job done—and that's where the B vitamins come in.

THE B VITAMINS

There are two main enzymes responsible for this homocysteine-clearing process. If an enzyme is a key that makes a certain metabolic process happen, a cofactor is grease in the lock—an enzyme turbobooster. The B vitamins are cofactors for the enzymes that foster this homocysteine-clearing process. So taking the appropriate B vitamins to supercharge those enzymes can help to compensate for an inherited inefficiency in clearing homocysteine naturally.

Which B vitamins work?

The B vitamin **folate,** or **folic acid,** is often in the news because it's our best prevention against neural tube birth defects. The March of Dimes recommends that women who are pregnant or trying to get pregnant take up to 800 micrograms a day for the duration of their pregnancy. In fact, this vitamin is so important that the FDA mandated that all bread products must now have folic acid added to them, in the same way that vitamins A and D are added to milk. Happily, folic acid also contributes to the fight against coronary heart disease by acting as a cofactor for one of the enzymes that removes homocysteine from the bloodstream. Interestingly, since the FDA mandate, the average blood homocysteine level has decreased dramatically in the United States.

Vitamin B_6, or pyridoxine, is the cofactor for the other enzyme that helps to clear homocysteine from the blood.

Treating High Homocysteine

The B vitamins are widely available in foods. Folate can be found in dark, leafy green vegetables like spinach, collard greens, swiss chard, kale, and broccoli. Orange juice is also a good source. B_6 can be found in bananas and peanuts. Since homocysteine is produced when the body is digesting meat, diets to control it often include a reduction in the amount of animal protein consumed. If a patient eats a lot of meat, we often ask that she cut back before she starts B vitamins. It's always wise to stop a bad habit instead of adding another pill to your daily regimen to compensate for it.

Much of the time, diet is not enough to control a severe homocysteine problem, so your doctor may suggest that you supplement your diet with these B vitamins.

There are two ways to treat a high homocysteine problem with B vitamins. Since there are primarily two different enzyme deficiencies that might be responsible for the problem, one treatment choice is to figure out which enzyme deficiency you have. To do this, we increase doses of one of the B vitamin supplements and retest your blood to see what—if anything—is working. It's time-consuming, and you'll spend a lot of money on homocysteine blood tests. The other alternative, since there's little real downside to taking multiple B vitamins, is to cover all bases and go for a vitamin B combination right off the bat. For about 80 percent of people with high homocysteine, this generalized approach will work fine. In fact, the supplement industry has come out with a number of "high homocysteine" tablets.

As you know, you shouldn't take any supplement without consulting with your doctor, and this a good example of the reasons why. You may need a higher dose of folic acid to correct your problem than the dose you can get from one of these combination pills. Because a high dose of folic acid is potentially dangerous unless it's taken under close medical supervision, it's illegal to sell any dose larger than 1 gram without a prescription. So talking to your doctor before pursuing this therapy is not only recommended, but necessary.

WHAT TO WATCH OUT FOR

There are two things to be careful about when you're treating high levels of homocysteine with B vitamins. The first is that high doses of B_6 can cause something called a **permanent peripheral neuropathy**, which is a numbness in the fingers and toes. This was discovered years ago, when physicians were using high doses of B_6 to help control menstrual pain. It happens when you take a lot—usually over 500 milligrams a day. So we don't suggest that our patients take more than 250 milligrams a day.

The other problem that comes up is that folic acid can mask the changes that occur on a standard blood test that might alert your doctor to a disease called pernicious anemia, which can cause serious—and permanent—neurological damage. This disease generally occurs in older people, and it's usually a fairly easy disease to diagnose and treat. But since the folic acid conceals it on the blood test, it can go dangerously undiagnosed and untreated as a result. The FDA knows that folic acid has this effect, which is why it's not possible to buy megadoses of folic acid—they want you to be medically supervised if you're going to be taking this vitamin at a level that can mask this anemia. I test my patients on high doses of folic acid for pernicious anemia (using a special test, called a methylmalonic acid test) at least once a year.

The treatment for pernicious anemia is actually B_{12}, which is one of the reasons this particular B vitamin joins the others in our cocktail. The theory is that by putting the B_{12} in the cocktail, you sidestep the danger by packaging the cure with the folic acid, the potential cause of the problem. The problem

SUPPLEMENT PLAN #3:
THE HOMOCYSTEINE SOLUTION PLAN

2 micrograms of folate, 250 milligrams of B_6, and 10,000 units of B_{12}

- *These doses must be guided by your physician. Some people require more folate and some less, and all require medical monitoring when taking B vitamins at this dose level.*

❗ Possibly Harmful: Red Yeast Rice

In China, this supplement has been used for thousands of years to treat coronary heart disease and is actually the base for one of the most widely used statin drugs, lovastatin. It may lower cholesterol, but it might also be hepatoxic, which means it can cause liver damage. There simply haven't been enough studies on this herb to know for sure, so I recommend that my patients avoid it.

Another basic issue with supplements in general and this one in particular: You just don't know what's in it. There's no federal regulation of these supplements, and quality control is notoriously bad. Citrinin is a toxic by-product of fermentation, and monacolins are the beneficial, cholesterol-lowering element. In 2001, a study was done on nine commercial preparations of red yeast rice. Very low levels of the cholesterol-lowering monacolins were found in the nine commercial products they tested, and the toxic citrinin was found in six of them. In the best-case scenario, nothing happens—no benefit, but no loss, either. In the worst-case scenario, you may actually be taking a toxic substance.

Until better studies are done and the preparation of this supplement is better regulated, I recommend that my patients avoid it.

---

with this theory is that the cause of pernicious anemia is an inability to absorb B_{12} from the digestive system. So when we're treating pernicious anemia, we either have to use huge doses of B_{12} orally, or we give it intramuscularly, by shot. So I'm not entirely convinced that adding a little bit of B_{12} to the cocktail will actually head this pernicious anemia problem off at the pass. I include it because the results of a prominent European study showed that the three Bs together were the most effective combination in lowering homocysteine.

11

MAKING (AND MAINTAINING) A LIFELONG COMMITMENT TO YOUR HEART

As you have now seen, heart attacks and coronary artery disease are largely *preventable*. With the right nutrition, exercise, medication (when indicated), and supplements, combined with other heart-healthy habits like avoiding cigarette smoke and maintaining a healthy weight, you can actually change your cardiac destiny and reverse the course of this disease.

With that goal in mind, over the course of this book we've explored the ways you can ensure that you're getting the most precise diagnosis and therapy paths possible. So now that you're on the right Nutrition, Exercise, Medication (if necessary), and Supplement Plans for your personal Cardiac Fingerprint, the only question outstanding is how you will maintain those great results. You can't stop now—your journey has only just begun. Preventing a heart attack, especially for those of you at high risk, must be a *lifelong* pursuit.

GET REGULAR CHECKUPS

We've found over and over again that one-size-fits-all recommendations don't work. The same is true when it comes to maintaining the terrific results you've achieved. Those great results came as a result of our new ability to individualize treatment plans to fit your metabolic imbalances. Going forward, you will have to play an active role in partnering with your doctor to customize your maintenance program to fit your needs as they evolve.

So the first and most important Prescription for heart-health maintenance is to maintain a good working relationship with your doctor—and don't miss your regular checkups!

It's essential, especially in the first year of your treatment, for you to be retested frequently and to stay in close touch with your doctor so he can track your progress and tweak your therapy, if needed. Not everyone responds the same way to the same things, and it's important that your treatment continue to be as tailor made for you as it can be.

How often should you be retested? Here's a useful yardstick: Medicare has approved payment for many of these tests five times in the first year and then once annually for people with appropriate diagnoses. If you've implemented significant therapeutic changes, whether those are changes in your medication or in your lifestyle, I recommend that you be retested every 3 to 4 months to determine whether those changes are working.

As the lifestyle changes you've made turn into habits and the drug therapies (if you're on any) begin to work, your numbers will improve. And once your new blood tests show that you've achieved the results you wanted to achieve and have reached the goal numbers set by your doctor, then you only need to be tested once a year unless something changes.

CONTINUING MEDICATION

As I've said before, the best combination therapy of all is the right medication combined with the right lifestyle. Even if the medication therapy you're on seems to be doing wonders on its own, you'll also want to implement the right diet and exercise program for your metabolic type. This will not only substantially improve the results you see from the medication, but it's better for your overall health.

Eventually, your commitment to these lifestyle changes may also mean that you can talk to your doctor about lowering the dose of your drug.

If you've instituted real and substantial lifestyle changes and your blood-test results are showing great improvement, you're probably wondering when it's appropriate to start either reducing the dose of your medication or backing away from it entirely. Clearly, this is something that you're going to have to decide in partnership with your doctor, but here are some basic guidelines.

- Have you lost a significant amount of excess body weight?
- Have you made substantial improvements in your diet?
- Have you maintained an exercise program for at least 3 months?
- Do you feel confident that you're able to maintain these changes for the rest of your life?

Have you lost a significant amount of excess body weight?

Obviously, this question is only pertinent if you were overweight to begin with. And it's impossible for me to determine here how much weight loss is enough— it depends on the size you were when you started! For instance, a 6-pound weight loss might be very "significant" for a woman who weighs 100 pounds, while a 240-pound man might have to lose a little bit more to see a difference in his metabolic marker numbers. But don't underestimate the power of even a slight weight loss! It's one of the biggest myths out there that someone who's 40 pounds overweight has to lose 39 to see any changes at all—even a slight weight loss can make a huge difference in your blood tests. So 6 pounds, even in a big guy, is more than enough to see some of these genes stop expressing themselves.

Have you made substantial improvements in your diet?

This is unquestionably linked to the question above, but it's worth a separate entry.

If you were overweight and have lost the excess fat, congratulations. But *how* you lost it can be as important as the fact that you did. Did you lose the weight healthfully? In other words, did you starve yourself or eat only cabbage soup for months? Or did you gradually learn to reconfigure your diet and exercise regimens so that you were burning more calories than you ate? Unhealthy and crash diets can put a lot of strain on your body and may prevent you from getting the nutrients you need—in fact, some weight-loss programs can hurt more than they help!

It's been proven that people who lose weight gradually and sensibly are more likely to keep it off, and I want this to be a lifelong change for you.

Those people who haven't ever been overweight aren't out of the woods either. It's a major misconception that your body mass index is the only indication of whether or not your diet needs to improve. If you're eating a bag of potato chips every day or a pint of ice cream every night, you need to rethink your diet, even if you're not overweight. There are tons of skinny people walking around with astronomical triglycerides and insulin levels—ticking time bombs, even though they look great in a bathing suit!

For optimal cardiac results, I strongly recommend a healthy, well-balanced diet that's rich in fruits, vegetables, soy protein, and whole grains—and most importantly, one that's specifically targeted to your particular metabolic profile.

Have you maintained an exercise program for at least 3 months?

Exercise can be as powerful a medication as some of the best cardiac drugs on the market. The results are only as good as your last workout, though, so it's essential that you maintain your new program consistently.

You may also find that your workout is getting easier the more you do it. You may find, for instance, that you're now cruising through the same 45-minute walk that left you huffing and puffing 3 months ago. Congratulations! That means you're getting fit! Make sure you're still getting the exercise your heart needs, though. You may have to increase your workout slightly to keep receiving those cardiovascular benefits. Use your target heart rate as your guide—as long as you're within your personal heart rate training zone for the prescribed amount of time, you're guaranteed to get the results you want.

Routine exercise is also important to maintain your hard-won weight loss. As I've mentioned, we conducted a study several years ago at Stanford University: People who lost weight simply by cutting calories gained it back within the year, but the people who lost weight by exercising kept the weight off.

Do you feel confident that you're able to maintain these changes for the rest of your life?

Making these changes is the hard part—it probably meant breaking a lot of bad habits and thinking about things in an entirely new way. The next step is in making a lifelong commitment to the changes you've made. Can you confidently say that you're going to be able to maintain them for the rest of your life?

I've found in my patients that the answer is generally yes. By and large, the lifestyle changes I've recommended are inexpensive, painless, and bring tremendous gains into the rest of their lives as well. I've never heard anybody wish they could gain the weight back, or lose their conditioning, or raise their cholesterol! The ever-improving numbers on the blood tests—coupled with the knowledge that the prospect of a heart attack or bypass surgery recedes as those numbers improve—is really a terrific motivator. So be realistic, but have confidence in yourself! You've made the best investment you could possibly make. Now you just have to commit to maintaining that investment over the long haul.

If you *have* made significant lifestyle changes—if you have lost a significant amount of body fat, made great improvements in your diet, maintained an exercise program for at least 3 months, and feel sure that you've made a lifelong commitment to your cardiac health, then a conversation with your doctor about medication is appropriate. Tell him that you want to begin to explore the idea of lowering the dose of the drug you're on, in order to see what effects it has on your blood-test results.

Note: If you and your doctor agree to reduce your medication, it is even more imperative that you make and keep your regular checkup appointments. Your doctor will want to ensure that your goal numbers are still holding on the lower dose and be able to make an immediate correction if they are not.

BE ALERT TO CHANGES

Once your metabolic marker numbers are fairly stable, getting retested once a year should be fine, *as long as everything else in your life has stayed the same.* You should be retested immediately if there is any kind of serious emotional or physical change in your life, because any kind of radical change might require us to rethink a therapy

> Get retested immediately if you experience any kind of serious emotional or physical change in your life.

path. Some of the changes you might want to watch out for include emotional turmoil at home or at work, a weight gain, the onset of menopause, or any other new medical conditions that might have an effect.

- Have you experienced serious emotional changes?
- Have you gained weight?
- Are you experiencing the onset of menopause?
- Have you been diagnosed with any new medical conditions or begun any new medication therapies?

Have you experienced serious emotional changes?

Don't underestimate the power of the mind to alter the body. I've seen serious disturbances in blood-test results after a patient has experienced some emotional trauma in his work or home life.

In many cases, there are explanations for this. Lots of people gain weight when they lose their jobs, for instance—they're spending more time at home and may be eating more to combat depression. A new stressful job might mean that you have a lot less time to exercise. A divorce might mean more takeout, and a death in the family might mean that you're suddenly too grief stricken or busy with new responsibilities to get to the gym.

When you stop eating healthily and exercising, even if that's not accompanied by a weight gain, your lipid numbers will show those unhealthy lifestyle changes very quickly. It's important that we get those numbers back under control immediately—jeopardizing your health isn't going to make your emotional condition any better. So if I hear that one of my patients has gone through some emotional turmoil recently—even if he hasn't gained weight—I ask him to come in for a test, and I'd advise you to consider the same.

Have you gained weight?

As you well know by now, I believe that maintaining a proper weight is one of the most important ways to maintain a healthy metabolic profile.

In fact, this is one of the most useful gauges I have in measuring the success of a patient's maintenance. Usually, if her weight is staying the same (and within healthy parameters), her metabolic profiles look good, too. An increase in weight is a first sign that something is going wrong.

And it doesn't need to be a lot of weight, either. One of my patients gained 4 pounds in 3 months. When I expressed concern about it, he tried to laugh me off. "Relax! It's just 4 pounds, Doc!" he said. He stopped laughing when I showed him how dramatically even that minor gain had affected his blood work: Those 4 pounds were enough to raise his small LDLs significantly, turning him from an LDL pattern A to a dangerous pattern B. Chastened, he stepped up his exercise and lost the pounds.

If someone gains weight, I'll retest him and rethink his individualized set of programs based on these results—and I'll want to have a conversation with that patient to see what's precipitated the sudden lifestyle change. Is there something in your life, some emotional trouble like the ones we've described above, that's causing you to eat more and exercise less? Have you picked up a seemingly innocuous habit (like an oatmeal cookie with your lunch a couple of times a week) that's getting you into trouble? You may want to keep a food record for a couple of days to see if something has changed without your conscious realization. Or you just may need to renew your commitment to getting and staying healthy.

Are you experiencing the onset of menopause?

Women will want to notify their doctors when they begin to go through menopause. As I've mentioned at various points throughout the book, reduced estrogen levels may have dramatic effects on your metabolic condition.

As a woman goes through menopause, we usually see a change in her standard cholesterol numbers; her LDL goes up as her HDL goes down. And the Advanced Metabolic Markers change as well: HDL2b takes a hit as her HDL levels drop, and the small LDL trait may begin to express itself.

In the past, if you were at high risk for coronary heart disease, we'd automatically recommend that you talk to your gynecologist about hormone therapy, but recent studies have made that a much more complicated and difficult choice. What I will say is this: Menopause is a time in your life when it's important to really pay attention to your metabolic issues. This is a time when many of these nasty genetic tendencies begin to express themselves in women, and you want to do everything you can to prevent them from doing so.

One way to do this is to focus on lifestyle issues. For instance, postmenopausal women have a tendency to gain weight more easily than they did before menopause, so that's something to watch out for. In fact, this is a good time to review all your lifestyle risk factors to see if there's anything you can change to improve your risk profile.

If your Advanced Metabolic Markers begin to show that you have elevated Lp(a) after the onset of menopause, you may want to be more aggressive, because this marker increases risk so drastically. One of the ways to combat this is by taking hormone therapy. So if you have a strong family history of coronary heart disease (a first-degree relative) and elevated Lp(a) with no other contraindications, you and your doctor may want to further explore the possibility of hormone therapy.

Have you been diagnosed with any new medical conditions or has your doctor prescribed any new medications?

The body is a series of connected systems, and when anything changes in one of those systems, it can have a truly profound effect on the others.

We've seen examples of this throughout the book; diabetes, for instance, has come up over and over again. This disease, although it is not a heart condition, is directly and inextricably linked to coronary artery disease—the two cannot be separated. And there are other medical conditions, even conditions that may appear to be unrelated to your heart, that have consequences on your blood work. So if you've been diagnosed with any other medical condition since your last metabolic marker test, you should absolutely be sure to let the doctor who's managing your lipids know.

This is especially true if you've begun taking any new medication. A beta-blocker may aggravate a high-triglyceride issue, some antidepressants can change lipid metabolism, and some AIDS medications may exacerbate existing coronary conditions. Your doctors can manage your medications so that you're getting the maximum amount of benefit for the least amount of risk, but you have to take the responsibility of reporting any changes immediately.

WHAT IF MY RESULTS SUDDENLY GO HAYWIRE?

Pay attention if your blood-test results suddenly change in radical and unexpected ways. If this happens and your doctor recommends that you be tested again, do so immediately.

It's not anything to get alarmed about; it may just be a problem with the lab or some physiological anomaly you're manifesting that month or even on that particular testing day. But I wouldn't suggest that you write it off automatically, either, especially if the fluctuation is significant. The standard lipid tests and these Advanced Metabolic Markers are good indicators, not only for coronary heart disease, but for other problems as well. Seeing a sudden abnormal change in blood-test results may indicate an early underlying disease state. For instance, I've caught a few patients in the early stages of cancer when I was tipped off by a sudden and otherwise inexplicable fluctuation in their metabolic marker results. Of course, aberrant results may just be aberrations, and most of the time that's all they are, but it's worth a retest to make sure that they're not signaling something else.

WHAT WILL CHANGE AS I AGE?

Will all this good work naturally fall apart as you get older? My answer is an emphatic *no!*

Contrary to popular belief, atherosclerosis isn't a natural process. It drives me crazy that people assume that coronary artery disease is an inevitable outcome of age—it's not, especially when you can diagnose the factors that contribute to it and treat those factors early, as we now can!

A 70-year-old *should* have perfectly immaculate arteries. It's important to remember that aging is more than the number of years you spend on the planet—it's what you do while you're here. The lighter the burden you put on your arteries, the younger they'll be, no matter what your chronological age. That means watching your diet, getting regular exercise, avoiding cigarette smoke, maintaining a healthy weight, seeing your doctor regularly, and taking your medications as they're prescribed to you.

One thing to watch out for: As people age, they tend to slow down. Sometimes this means that they gain weight—a big no-no for all the reasons we've discussed. But I'd like to discourage any reduction in activity, even if it's not accompanied by weight gain, as older people often experience a reduction in appetite as well. The cardiac (and overall) benefits of exercise extend beyond weight control, and every effort should be made to maintain a regular fitness regimen. Talk to your doctor if you have physical limitations; he can suggest accommodations so you can keep active.

KEEP READING!

One of the most important things you can do to optimize your cardiac health in the future is to keep an eye on new developments in the scientific literature.

As you know, we have crossed an important threshold, so things are changing very fast in this field. There are any number of new developments on the horizon that may have profound, life-extending ramifications on your cardiac health.

Now, this doesn't mean that you need to start combing the abstracts in the *New England Journal of Medicine*. It simply means that you pay attention to new studies reported in the popular media and that you follow up on them with your health practitioner. If you hear about something you think might be relevant, make a note to ask your doctor about it.

Your doctor may tell you a study was badly designed, or done in too small a population, or that the risks of an experimental therapy path outweigh the benefits. That's perfectly okay! It's wise to take everything you see on television or read in magazines or on the Internet with a grain of salt, and it's essential to trust your physician to interpret this information on your behalf. If you feel that your concerns aren't being heard, you're also welcome to pursue a second opinion. The more responsibility you take for your own prevention and care, the better that care will be. It is possible for the diligent patient to get a jump on the medicine of the future.

IN CONCLUSION

Groundbreaking advancements in the field of cardiology are coming at a fast and furious pace, and it's a tremendously exciting time to be researching and treating patients in this field as a result. I will tell you this: The trend toward the individualization of diagnosis and treatment—something we've explored at great length in this book—is here to stay.

With these Advanced Metabolic Markers, you and your doctor now have the tools to more accurately diagnose your risk level than ever before—dictating how aggressively you should act to treat your disease, and allowing you to treat the factors that put you at risk long before they've done the kind of damage that necessitates more invasive treatments, like surgery.

These tools also lead us to much more specific, targeted therapy paths than ever before. We're no longer treating 100 percent of our patients the same way, in the hopes that we catch the percentage who will actually benefit from that particular treatment. We can now fine-tune our recommendations to an astonishing degree, optimizing every bite you take, every step you run, and every pill you swallow, so that you're able to make the best choices for your personal combination of metabolic abnormalities, genetic tendencies, and risk factors.

Coronary heart disease doesn't have to be relentlessly progressive. You *can* outwit your genes. A brand new day has dawned already, and the future is bright with new hope and real choices for those whose lives are affected by coronary heart disease.

AFTERWORD

METABOLIC SYNDROME

Undoubtedly you have heard about the epidemic of obesity sweeping the Western world. It has been in all the newspapers and news magazines. Why is this "suddenly" happening and how is it related to the topics in *Before the Heart Attacks*? Is it something you should worry about?

First, it is true. The country is getting fatter. Look at the maps of the United States in Figures 1 and 2. They represent the United States in 1985 and 2002. The charts show the percentage of people in each state deemed to be obese by virtue of a BMI (see page 322 for a definition) greater than 30. This expanding pattern looks like some virulent infectious disease laying waste to large numbers of Americans. For some reason, obesity is becoming commonplace. But who among us is getting fat?

Well, one thought is that it is actually a result of the success of medicine in keeping people alive longer. Perhaps it is the older people. Is it because these elderly people can't exercise much because of arthritis, but can afford good and plentiful food and wine, that they are socking on the calories and getting fat? This seems to make sense but it is *wrong*. It is actually the *younger* people who are getting fatter faster than the older folks. The increase in obesity is 45 percent in people aged 60 to 69 years and 70 percent in young people aged 18 to 29 years! Well, is it because young people are couch potatoes and are playing too many video games sitting in front of TVs? While inactivity certainly plays a role, a bigger culprit is a change in American eating habits.

The emphasis on low-fat foods has succeeded in leading the country away from diets high in fat, but there has been a downside. A focus on low-fat foods has resulted in higher sugar consumption by the average American citizen.

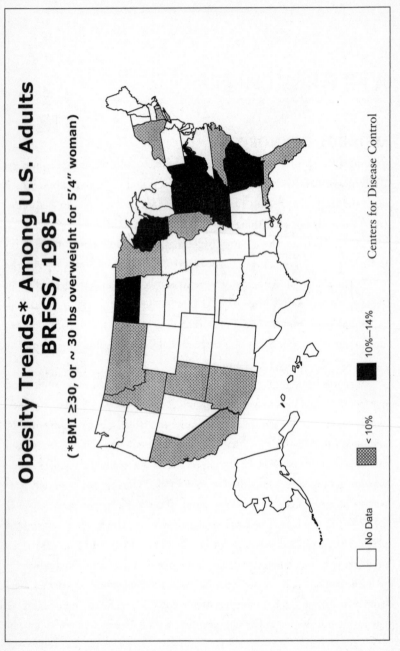

Obesity Trends* Among U.S. Adults
BRFSS, 1985

(*BMI ≥30, or ~ 30 lbs overweight for 5'4" woman)

No Data   < 10%   10%—14%

Centers for Disease Control

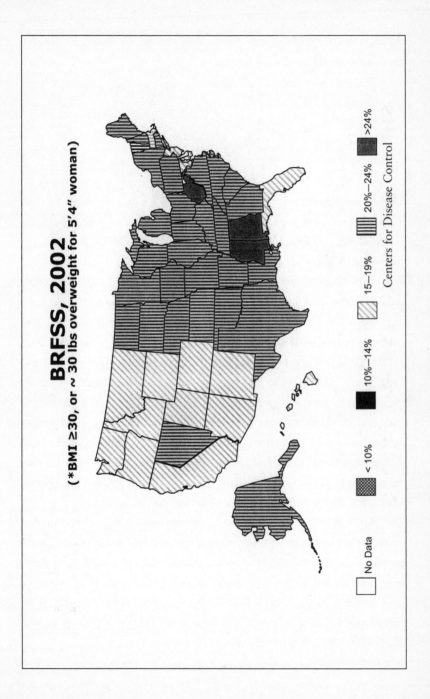

What do you think? How much sugar does the average American eat each day? Does the average American eat:

a) 1 tablespoon
b) ⅓ cup
c) ¼ pound
d) ½ pound

The answer is that the typical American now eats, on average, more than half a pound of simple sugar each day! Go to the supermarket, weigh out half a pound of sugar, and imagine eating that each and every day. Do you think you would put on a few pounds of body fat?

So how does this fit in with the "metabolic syndrome" and what exactly is the "metabolic syndrome"? There are a variety of ways to answer this question. Medically, the metabolic syndrome is a collection of factors that contribute to heart disease risk and include the ones you are familiar with, such as high blood pressure, high blood fats, and a proclivity to diabetes. But it also includes a number of other factors that you have read about in *Before the Heart Attacks*: an abundance of small LDL, elevated blood insulin levels, and a tendency for blood to clot. Many of these factors have an inherited component and tend to run in families. Thus, the metabolic syndrome is simply a collection of factors that increases heart disease risk that tend to go along with an overweight status. Currently about 25 percent of the American population has the metabolic syndrome. That's 47 million people!

This is all very interesting from a medical standpoint, but the really fascinating story is why this happens to so many people. If it were so bad, these people would die off, not get a chance to procreate and pass the gene on to their children, and the problem would become much smaller. Whenever there is an inherited disorder that is deadly, yet very common, there must be some benefit to it. Otherwise it would not be common. What could possibly be beneficial about the ability to get *fat*?

Well, this gets us to the "thrifty gene" concept proposed by Dr. James

Neel in 1962. He suggested that a series of genes exist that help humans survive in a primitive environment. In other words, if you lived in Africa 50,000 years ago and could kill an animal and gorge yourself on all the animal fat, and you had a set of genes that allowed your body to store fat up rapidly and efficiently, and that perhaps made you eat a bit more than you needed, this could be a real survival benefit because you may not get anything to eat for the next few days. For men, this would help sock on the muscle, look good to the women, and increase your chance of attracting a mate and procreating, thus passing these "survival" genes on to your lucky offspring. For women, these genes would help maintain body fat, which is necessary to menstruate, get pregnant, and help the tribe survive. In other words, genes that help you sock on the fat help you survive in an environment that does not have easily available diet calories.

Now think of it this way. For 150,000 years humans have benefited from these "thrifty genes"; but it is only in the past 200 years that the human population has had enough and even an excess number of diet calories that these survival genes are turning into deadly genes. It's of interest to note that in countries that do not have an excess of calories, the metabolic syndrome is not much of a problem. Perhaps our modern lifestyle is killing off all the genetically "normal" fat people and letting the mutant thin people survive?

With all this in mind, the cure for the metabolic syndrome is both simple and complex. Simply, exercise, eat right, and lose excess body fat. The complexity is, how do you do it in this high-stress, sedentary day and age? It is difficult to run around on foot and hunt your food each day but easy to go to the vending machine and purchase high-calorie foods with an easy flick of the finger. As mentioned in *Before the Heart Attacks,* it is best to exercise one hour per day, seven days per week to obtain reasonable benefit from exercise. It is also best to go to bed hungry. The concept of having a late-night snack may be particularly harmful.

The issue of how much exercise is necessary to burn off calories may best be illustrated by the type and amount of exercise it would take the author of this book to burn off the calories from one fast-food restaurant hamburger.

Activity	Time (minutes)
Martial arts	42
Shoveling coal in a coal mine	60
Moderate jogging	60
Skiing downhill	70
Playing golf (carrying clubs)	93

Okay, so a lot of this is linked to being overweight. How do you determine if you are overweight? Is it simply how much you weigh? One tool is the calculation of body mass index (BMI), as explained in *Before the Heart Attacks*. The BMI is simply weight (in kilograms) divided by height (in meters) squared (BMI = weight (kg)/height (meter)^2. This is a very useful research tool to use in studies of large groups of people, but can be misleading in individual patients. The US Adult Treatment Panel guidelines recommend simply measuring your waist (waist circumference). According to the US Adult Treatment Panel, if you are a woman with a waist greater that 35 inches, you are overweight. Does this sound right to you? Well, what if you are 5'2'' inches tall with a waist of 40 inches, or 6'2'' tall with a waist of 40 inches? This would certainly represent two very different-looking people.

The World Health Organization has done one better, and it relates to the "gut-to-butt" ratio that we used at Stanford University in weight loss studies many years ago. The concept is simple: Measure the circumference of the gut (waist) and the circumference of the butt (hips), and see which is bigger. This helps determine if you have body fat in the typical apple or pear shape. The apple shape is a typical "male" body fat pattern, with the waist bigger than the hips. This body fat pattern is particularly nasty, as it is strongly linked to increased heart disease risk. The pear shape is used to describe a typical "female" body fat pattern, where more of the fat is carried around the stomach area.

The World Health Organization has refined this to the "waist-to-hip" ratio. It also sounds better than the "gut-to-butt" ratio. If this ratio is >1.0 in a man or >0.8 in a woman, you are overweight. Great. This takes care of how tall you are, but where do you measure your waist and hips? Well, the waist can be measured at the level of the belly button, and the hips at—guess where—the widest point. This makes a lot of practical sense since almost every woman can judge if she is gaining or losing weight by how she fits into her clothing, and men will often note that they need to take in another notch in their belt when they are losing weight.

In *Before the Heart Attacks* you learned the importance of high-density lipoprotein (HDL), different types of HDL, and the concept of reverse cholesterol transport. This process, which helps remove cholesterol that forms blockages in the arteries, relies heavily on a protein attached to the HDL called apoprotein AI. These proteins dive in and out of the spherical HDL, much like an old-fashioned sea serpent illustrated undulating in and out of the ocean. Believe it or not, this story is linked to Milan, Italy.

In 1980 a group of people belonging to the same family tree living in a town north of Milan (Limone sur Garda) was discovered to have low HDL cholesterol (averaging about 20 mg /dl instead of the more normal average of 45 mg/dl). These people should have been ravaged by heart disease, yet coronary heart disease is virtually unheard of and they all seem to live long, healthy lives. What a paradox! Low HDL cholesterol and freedom from heart disease. How could this possibly be explained?

Of further interest is the ability of medical researchers to identify a gene responsible for this paradox called the Apo AI Milano gene. These people have a genetic difference that produced a unique type of apoprotein A that, because it looks a lot like a corkscrew, protects those who have it from heart disease. Its inheritance can be traced back to a man named Giovanni Pomaroli and a woman named Rosa Giovaneli, who procreated all the offspring who now carry this productive genetic difference. Fascinating, but how can it possibly help you? Even if you marry into the family, it might help your children but the gene can't be transferred to you. Or can it?

In the 1980s medical researchers were investigating if manipulation of HDL could benefit heart disease patients. Of course, before any new therapy is tried in humans, it is tried in mice first. Dr. Eddie Rubin at the University of California, Berkeley, created a bunch of artificial HDL particles in a test tube, and over the course of several weeks injected them into the bloodstream of mice that had particularly blocked arteries. He showed that with the artificial increase in blood HDL levels, the heart disease in the mice was dramatically reversed. Terrific, but will this require weekly injections? Well, his next step was to isolate the human gene responsible for making apoprotein A and HDL, affix it to a virus, and inject the virus and DNA of the good apoprotein A into mice with heart disease. As you might guess, the human DNA was active, produced vast quantities of apoprotein A, and increased HDL dramatically. This resulted in a remarkable reversal of atherosclerosis in the mice.

The real question is, when can we treat humans as well as we treat mice? Well, it's not so far away. Initial experiments have already been conducted in humans, and the day is not too far away when humans with heart disease can receive either an infusion of HDL made in a test tube or a gene that will result in dramatically increased HDL circulating in the blood that will mean freedom from heart disease. Until that time, it is only reasonable to do all one can to increase HDL through appropriate lifestyle (such as proper diet, exercise, and weight control), and if necessary, take medications delivered under a physician's supervision, such as niacin and fenofibrate, and drugs in the pipeline called CETP inhibitors.

SELECTED BIBLIOGRAPHY

1. **Factors other than LDL-C are powerful markers of heart disease risk.**

Brunzell, J. D., Chait, A., Albers, J. J., Foster, D. M., Failor, R. A., Bierman, E. L. Metabolic consequences of genetic heterogeneity of lipoprotein composition (lipoprotein heterogeneity). *American Heart Journal* 113 (1987): 583–587.

Krauss, R. M. The tangled web of coronary risk factors. *American Journal of Medicine* 90 (1991): 36S–41S.

Ross, R. The pathogenesis of atherosclerosis: a perspective for the 1990s. *Nature* 362 (1993): 801–809.

Steinberg, D. Beyond cholesterol. Modifications of low-density lipoprotein that increase its atherogenicity. *New England Journal of Medicine* 320 (1989): 915–921.

Superko, H. R. Beyond LDL-C reduction. *Circulation* 94 (1996): 2351–2354.

Tribble, D. L., van den Berg, J. J. M., Motchnik, P. A., Ames, B. N., Lewis, D. M., Chait, A., Krauss, R. M. Oxidative susceptibility of low density lipoprotein subfractions is related to their ubiquinol-10 and alpha-tocopherol content. *Proceedings of the National Academy of Sciences USA* 91 (1994): 1183–1187.

2. **Small LDL increases the risk of heart disease.**

Austin, M. A. Triglycerides, small, dense low-density lipoprotein, and the atherogenic lipoprotein phenotype. *Current Atherosclerosis Reports* 2[3] (May 2000): 200–207.

Austin, M. A., King, M. C., Vranizan, K. M., Krauss, R. M. Atherogenic lipoprotein phenotype. A proposed genetic marker for coronary heart disease risk. *Circulation* 82 (1990): 495–506.

Gardner, C. D., Fortmann, S. P., Krauss, R. M. Association of small low-density lipoprotein particles with the incidence of coronary artery disease in men and women. *JAMA* 276 (1996): 875–881.

Gofman, J. W., Young, W., Tandy, R. Ischemic heart disease, atherosclerosis and longevity. *Circulation* 34 (1966): 679–697.

Lamarche, B., Tchernof, A., Mauriege, P., Cantin, B., Dagenais, G. R., Lupien, P. J., Despres, J. P. Fasting insulin and apolipoprotein B levels and low-density lipoprotein particle size as risk factors for ischemic heart disease. *JAMA* 279 (1998): 1955–1961.

Nordestgaard, B. G., Wootton, R., Lewis, B. Selective retention of VLDL, IDL, and LDL in the arterial intima of genetically hyperlipidemic rabbits in vivo. Molecular size as a determinant of fractional loss from the intima-inner media. *Arteriosclerosis, Thrombosis, and Vascular Biology* 15 (1995): 534–542.

Stampfer, M. J., Krauss, R. M., Blanche, P. J., Holl, L. G., Sacks, F. M., Hennekens, C. H. A prospective study of triglyceride level, low density lipoprotein particle diameter, and risk of myocardial infarction. *JAMA* 276 (1996): 882–888.

Superko, H. R. The atherogenic lipoprotein profile. *Science and Medicine* 4 (1997): 36–45.

Vakkilainen, J., Makimattila, S., Seppala-Lindroos, A., Vehkavaara, S., Lahdenpera, S., Groop, P. H., Taskinen, M. R., Yki-Jarvinen, H. Endothelial dysfunction in men with small LDL particles. *Circulation* 102 (2000): 716–721.

3. **Treatment of small LDL is beneficial.**

Krauss, R. M., Lindgren, F. T., Williams, P. T., Kelsey, S. F., Brensike, J., Vranizan, K., Detre, K. M., Levy, R. I. Intermediate-density lipoproteins and progression of coronary artery disease in hypercholesterolaemic men. *Lancet* 2 (1987): 62–65.

Miller, B. D., Alderman, E. L., Haskell, W. L., Fair, J. M., Krauss, R. M. Predominance of dense low-density lipoprotein particles predicts angiographic benefit or therapy in the Stanford Coronary Risk Intervention project. *Circulation* 94 (1996): 2146–2153.

Superko, H. R. What can we learn about dense LDL and lipoprotein particles from clinical trials? *Current Opinion in Lipidology* 7 (1996): 363–368.

Superko, H. R., Krauss, R. M. Coronary artery disease regression. Convincing evidence for the benefit of aggressive lipoprotein management. *Circulation* 90 (1994): 1056–1069.

Zambon, A., Hokanson, J. E., Brown, B. G., Brunzell, J. D. Evidence for a new pathophysiological mechanism for coronary artery disease regression. *Circulation* 99 (1999): 1959–1964.

4. Lipids and diabetes

Austin, M. A, Mykkanen, L., Kuusisto, J., Edwards, K. L., Nelson, C., Haffner, S. M., Pyorala, K., Laakso, M. Prospective study of small LDLs as a risk factor for non-insulin dependent diabetes mellitus in elderly men and women. *Circulation* 92 (1995): 1770–1778.

Eckel, R. H., Wassef, M., Chait, A., et al. Diabetes and cardiovascular disease writing group II: pathogenesis of atherosclerosis in diabetes. *Circulation* 105 (2002): e138–e143.

Superko, H. R. Current and future trends in therapy for dyslipidemias. *Endocrine Practice* 3 (1997): 255–263.

5. Apolipoproteins

Brewer, H. B., Gregg, R. E., Hoeg, J. M., Fojo, S. S. Apolipoproteins and lipoproteins in human plasma: an overview. *Clinical Chemistry* 34 (1988): B4–B8.

Franceschini, G., Sirtori, C. R., Capurso, K. H., Weisgraber, K. H., Mahley, R. W. The A-I Milano apoprotein. I. Decreased high-density lipoprotein cholesterol levels with significant lipoprotein modifications and without clinical atherosclerosis in an Italian family. *Journal of Clinical Investigation* 66 (1980): 892–900.

Nissen, S.E. Tsunoda, T., Tuzcu, E. Murat, Schoenhagen, P., Cooper, C. J., Yasin, M., Eaton, G. M., Lauer, M. A. Sheldon, W. S., Grines, C. L., Halpern, S., Crowe, T., Blankenship, J. C., and Kerensky, R.. Effect of recombinant ApoA-I Milano on coronary atherosclerosis in patients with acute coronary syndromes: a randomized controlled trial. *JAMA* 290 (2003): 2292–2300.

Sniderman, A. D., Bergeron, J., Frohlich, J. Apolipoprotein B versus lipoprotein lipids: vital lessons from the AFCAPS/TexCAPS trial. *Canadian Medical Association Journal* 164 (2001): 44–47.

Sniderman, A. D., Cianflone, K. Measurement of apolipoproteins: time to improve the diagnosis and treatment of the atherogenic dyslipoproteinemias. *Clinical Chemistry* 42 (1996): 489–491.

6. Lp(a)

Maher, V. M. G., Brown, B. G., Marcovina, S., Hilger, L. A., Zhao, X. Q., Albers, J. J. Effects of lowering elevated LDL cholesterol on the cardiovascular risk of lipoprotein(a). *JAMA* 274 (1995): 1771–1774.

Scanu, A. Lipoprotein(a): a genetic risk factor for premature coronary heart disease. *JAMA* 267 (1992): 3326–3329.

7. Homocysteine

Appel, L. J., Miller, E. R., Ha Jee, S., Stolzenberg-Solomon, R., Lin, P. H., Erlinger, T., Nadeau, M. R., Shelhub, J. Effect of dietary patterns on homocysteine. *Circulation* 102 (2000): 852–857.

Chambers, J. C., Obeid, O. A., Refsum, H., Ueland, P., Hackett, D., Hooper, J., Turner, R. M., Thompson, S. G., Kooner, J. S. Plasma homocysteine concentrations and risk of coronary heart disease in UK Indian Asian and European men. *Lancet* 355 [9203] (2000): 523–527.

Dalery, K., Lussier, C. S., Shelhub, J., Davignon, J., Latour, Y., Genest, J. Jr. Homocysteine and coronary artery disease in French Canadian subjects: relation with vitamins B_{12}, B_6, pyridoxal phosphate, and folate. *American Journal of Cardiology* (75) 1995: 1107–1111.

Graham, I. M., Daly, L. E., Refsum, H. M., Robinson, K., Brattstrom, L. E., Ueland, P. M., Palma-Reis, R. J., Boers, G. H. J., Sheahan, R. G., Israelsson, B., Uiterwaal, C. S., Meleady, R., McMaster, D., Verhoef, P., Witteman, J., Rubba, P., Bellet, H., Wautrecht, J. C., de Valk, H. W., Sales, A. C., Parrot-Roulaud, F. M., Tan, K. S., Higgins, I., Garcon, D., Medrano, M. J., Candito, M., Evans, A. E., Andria, G. Plasma homocysteine as a risk factor for vascular disease. The European Concerted Action Project. *JAMA* 277 (1997): 1775–1781.

Hoogeveen, E. K., Kostense, P. J., Beks, P. J., Mackaay, A. J., Jakobs, C., Bouter, L. M., Heine, R. J., Stehouwer, C. D. Hyperhomocysteinemia is associated with an increased risk of cardiovascular disease, especially in non-insulin-dependent diabetes mellitus: a population based study. *Arteriosclerosis, Thrombosis, and Vascular Biology* 18 (1998): 133–138.

Jacques, P. F., Selhub, J., Bostom, A. G., Wilson, P. W., Rosenberg, I. H. The effect of folic acid fortification on plasma folate and total homocysteine concentrations. *New England Journal of Medicine* 34 (1999): 1449–1454.

8. Inflammation and hs-CRP

Festa, A., D'Agostino, R. Jr., Howard, G., et al. Chronic subclinical inflammation as part of the insulin resistance syndrome: the Insulin Resistance Atherosclerosis Study (IRAS). *Circulation* 10 (2000): 42–47.

Ridker, P. M. High-sensitivity C-reactive protein. *Circulation* 103 (2001): 1813–1818.

Ross, R. Atherosclerosis—an inflammatory disease. *New England Journal of Medicine* 340 (1999): 115–126.

9. Reverse cholesterol transport

Brown, G. B., Zhao, X. Q., Chait, A., Fisher, L. D., Cheung, M. C., Morse, J. S., Dowdy, A. A., Marino, E. K., Bolson, E. L., Alaupovic, P., Frohlich, J., Albers, J. J. Simvastatin and niacin, antioxidant vitamins, or the combination for the prevention of coronary disease. *New England Journal of Medicine* 345 (2001): 1583–1592.

Franceschini, G., Bondioli, A., Granata, D., Mercuri, V., Negri. M., Tosi, C., Sirtori, C. R. Reduced HDL2 levels in myocardial infarction patients without risk factors for atherosclerosis. *Atherosclerosis* 68 (1987): 213–219.

Laakso, M., Voutilainen, E., Pyorala, K., Sarlund, H. Association of low HDL and HDL2 cholesterol with coronary heart disease in noninsulin-dependent diabetics. *Arteriosclerosis* 5 (1985): 653–658.

Sviridov, D., Nestel, P. Dynamics of reverse cholesterol transport: protection against atherosclerosis. *Atherosclerosis* 161[2] (2002): 245–254.

10. Metabolic syndrome and obesity

Ford, E. S., Giles, W. H., Dietz, W. H. Prevalence of the metabolic syndrome among US adults. *JAMA* 287 (2002): 356–359.

Lakka, H. M., Laaksonen, D. E., Niskanen, L. K., et al. The metabolic syndrome and total and cardiovascular disease mortality in middle-aged men. *JAMA* 288 (2002): 2709–2716.

McGill, H. C., McMahan, C. A., Henderick, E. E., et al. Obesity accelerates the progression of coronary atherosclerosis in young men. *Circulation* 105 (2002): 2712–2718.

Mokdad, A. H., Serdula, M. K., Dietz, W. H., Bowman, B. A., Marks, J. S., Koplan, J. P. The spread of the obesity epidemic in the United States, 1991–1998. *JAMA* 282 (1999): 1519–1522.

Reaven, G. Metabolic syndrome. *Circulation* 106 (2002): 286–288.

Reaven, G. M., Ida Chen, Y. D., Jeppesen, J., Maheux, P., Krauss, R. M. Insulin resistance and hyperinsulinemia in individuals with small, dense low density lipoprotein particles. *Journal of Clinical Investigation* 92 (1993): 141–146.

Superko, H. R. Metabolic syndrome, in *The Heart,* edited by J. Willis Hurst, 2004.

11. Postprandial lipemia

Brown, D. F., Heslin, S. A., Doyle, J. T. Postprandial lipemia in health and in ischemic heart disease. *New England Journal of Medicine* 264 (1961): 733–737.

Superko, H. R., Krauss, R. M. Garlic powder, effect on plasma lipids, postprandial lipemia, LDL particle size, HDL subclass distribution, and Lp(a). *Journal of the American College of Cardiology* 35 (2000): 321–326.

Zilversmit, D. B. Atherogenesis: a postprandial phenomenon. *Circulation* 60 (1979): 473–485.

12. Diet

Dreon, D. M., Fernstrom, H., Miller, B., Krauss, R. M. Low density lipoprotein subclass patterns and lipoprotein response to a reduced-fat diet in men. *FASEB Journal* 8 (1994): 121–126.

Ginsberg, H., Olefsky, J., Farquhar, J., Reaven, G. M. Moderate ethanol ingestion and plasma triglyceride levels. A study in normal and hypertriglyceridemic persons. *Annals of Internal Medicine* 80 (1974): 143–149.

Knopp, R. H., Walden, C. E., Retzlaff, B. M., McCann, B. S., Dowdy, A. A., Albers, J. J., Gey, G. O., Cooper, M. N. Long-term cholesterol-lowering effects of 4 fat-restricted diets in hypercholesterolemic and combined hyperlipidemic men. The Dietary Alternatives Study. *JAMA* 278 [18] (1997): 1509–1515.

Krauss, R. M. Genetic, metabolic, and dietary influences on the atherogenic lipoprotein phenotype. Simopoulos, A.P. (ed): Genetic variation and dietary response. *World Review of Nutrition and Dietetics*. Basel, Karger 80 (1997): 22–43.

Krauss, R. M. Atherogenic lipoprotein phenotype and diet-gene interactions. *Journal of Nutrition* 131 (2001): 340S–343S.

Spiller, G. A., Jenkins, D. J. A., Cragen, L. N., Gates, J. E., Bosello, O., Berra, K., Rudd, C., Stevenson, M., Superko, H. R. Effect of a diet high in monounsaturated fat from almonds on plasma cholesterol and lipoproteins. *Journal of the American College of Nutrition* 11 (1992): 126–130.

Superko, H. R. Effects of acute and chronic alcohol consumption on postprandial lipemia in healthy normotriglyceridemic men. *American Journal of Cardiology* 69 (1992): 701–704.

Superko, H. R., Bortz, W., Williams, P. T., Albers, J. J., Wood, P. D. Effects of caffeinated and decaffeinated coffee on plasma lipoprotein cholesterol and apolipoproteins in men. *American Journal of Clinical Nutrition* 54 (1991): 599–605.

Superko, H. R., Myll, J., DiRicco, C., Williams, P., Bortz, W., Wood, P. D. Cessation of caffeinated coffee consumption reduces ambulatory blood pressure but not resting blood pressure in men. *American Journal of Cardiology* 73 (1994): 780–784.

Williams, P. T., Krauss, R. M., Kindel-Joyce, S., Dreon, D. M., Vranizan, K. M., Wood, P. D. Relationship of dietary fat, protein, cholesterol, and fiber intake to atherogenic lipoproteins in men. *American Journal of Clinical Nutrition* 44 (1986): 788–797.

Williams, P. T., Krauss, R. M., Vranizan, K. M., Wood, P. D. Changes in lipoprotein subfractions during diet-induced and exercise-induced weight loss in moderately overweight men. *Circulation* 81 (1990): 1293–1304.

13. Exercise

Superko, H. R. Exercise training, serum lipids and lipoprotein particles: Is there a change threshold? *Exercise and Sports in Science and Medicine* 23 (1991): 677–685.

Superko, H. R. Exercise and lipoprotein metabolism. *Journal of Cardiovascular Risk* 2 (1995): 310–315.

Williams, P. T., Krauss, R. M., Vranizan, K. M., Albers, J. J., Terry, R. B., Wood, P. D. Effects of exercise induced weight loss on low density lipoprotein subfractions in healthy men. *Arteriosclerosis* 9 (1989): 623–632.

Wood, P. D., Haskell, W. L. The effect of exercise on plasma high density lipoproteins. *Lipids* 14 (1979): 417–427.

Wood, P. D., Stefanick, M. L., Dreon, D. M., Frey-Hewitt, B., Garay, S. C., Williams, P. T., Superko, H. R., Fortmann, S. P., Albers, J. J., Vranizan, K. M., Ellsworth, N. M., Terry, R. B., Haskell, W. L. Changes in plasma lipids and lipoproteins during weight loss by dieting versus exercise in overweight men. *New England Journal of Medicine* 319 (1988): 1173–1179.

14. Medications

Brown, B. G., Zambon, A., Poulin, D., Rocha, A., Maher, V. M., Davis, J. W., Albers, J. J., Brunzell, J. D. Use of niacin, statins, and resins in patients with combined hyperlipidemia. *American Journal of Cardiology* 81[4A] (1998): 52B–59B.

Canner, P. L., Berge, K. G., Wenger, N. K., Stamler, J., Friedman, L., Prineas, R. J., Friedewald, W. Fifteen year mortality in coronary drug project patients: long-term benefit with niacin. *Journal of the American College of Cardiology* 8 (1986): 1245–1255.

Guyton, J. R., Goldberg, A. C., Kreisberg, R. A., Sprecher, D. L., Superko, H. R., O'Connor, C. M. Effectiveness of once-nightly dosing of extended release niacin alone and in combination for hypercholesterolemia. *American Journal of Cardiology* 82 (1998): 737–743.

Superko, H. R. Hypercholesterolemia and dyslipidemia. *Current Treatment Options in Cardiovascular Medicine* 2 (2000): 173–187.

Superko, H. R., Krauss, R. M. Differential effects of nicotinic acid in subjects with different LDL subclass patterns. *Atherosclerosis* 95 (1992): 69–76.

Superko, H. R., Krauss, R. M., Haskell, W. L. Stanford Coronary Risk Intervention Project Investigators. Association of lipoprotein subclass distribution with use of selective and non-selective beta-blocker medications in patients with coronary heart disease. *Atherosclerosis* 101 (1993): 1–8.

INDEX

from food sources, 285
ratings of, 284

T

Target heart rate
  benefits of using, 219–21, 223, 309–10
  calculating, 217–18
  purpose of, 215–17
TC, 47–48
Testing. *See* Screening tests
Thallium exercise test, 103
Thiazolidine-diones, <u>280</u>
Thrifty gene concept, explaining obesity, 140–41
Thrombosis, 9–10, 285–86
Thyroid disease, affecting lipids, 243
Total cholesterol (TC), meaning of, 47–48
Trans fats, 124–25, <u>124</u>
Treadmill tests, 102–3, 212
Tricor, 277
Triglycerides
  diet affecting, 169, 180
  exercise removing, 208–9
  HDL and, 237
  high
    Antioxidant Defense Plan for, <u>291</u>, 292
    Better-Carbohydrate, Lower-Carbohydrate Diet for, 193
    bile acid–binding resins contraindicated with, 262
    Fish Oil Rx Plan for, 297
    Heavyweight Plan for, <u>265</u>, 266
  high-fat meal affecting, 151–52
  increased by
    alcohol, <u>132–33</u>, 184
    carbohydrates, 126, 128
    medications, <u>246</u>
    sugars, 179–80, 192
  understanding levels of, 50–51, 94
Type A/type B personalities, coronary heart disease risk and, 36–37

U

Ulcers, peptic, niacin contraindicated for, 276
Uric acid, niacin increasing, 270

V

Vacations, dietary splurges on, 152
Vasoconstriction, factors increasing, 11
Vasodilators, avoiding, with niacin, 274–75
Vasoreactivity, 10–11, 258–59, 279
VEAPS, 295
Ventricles, 4
Vertex male-pattern baldness, predicting coronary heart disease risk, 26–27
Very low-density lipoprotein (VLDL), 47–48, 236, 237, 266
Vitamin B$_6$
  food sources of, 303
  for lowering homocysteine, 303, <u>304</u>
  peripheral neuropathy from, 304
Vitamin B$_{12}$, in Homocysteine Solution Plan, 304–5, <u>304</u>
Vitamin C
  in Antioxidant Defense Plan, 295–96
  heart protection from, <u>162</u>
  niacin and, 295
Vitamin E
  in Antioxidant Defense Plan, 294–95
  heart protection from, <u>162</u>
  niacin and, 295
  smokers and, 293
Vitamin E Atherosclerosis Prevention Study (VEAPS), 295
Vitamins, function of, 283
VLDL, 47–48, 236, 237, 266

W

Waist circumference, indicating overweight, 33
Water drinking, during exercise, <u>215</u>
Weight gain
  with aging, 315
  retesting metabolic markers after, 312
Weight loss
  for conversion to LDL pattern A, 231
  determining calorie requirements for, 142–44, <u>143</u>, <u>144</u>, 157